THE OFFICIAL YMCA GUIDE

You & Me Baby

Susan L. Regnier, National Coordinator
You & Me, Baby Program
YMCA of the USA

MEADOWBROOK BOOKS
18318 Minnetonka Boulevard
Deephaven, Minnesota 55391

Library of Congress Cataloging in Publication Data

Regnier, Susan L., 1956-
    You & me, baby.

    Bibliography: p. 179
    Includes index.
    1. Pregnancy. 2. Exercise for women. 3. Infants—Care and hygiene. 4. Exercise for children. I. Title. II. Title: You and me, baby.
RG558.7.R44   1984   618.2'4   83-23826
ISBN 0-88166-017-5 (paperback)

10 9 8 7 6 5 4 3 2 1
Printed in the United States of America

© 1983, 1984 by Susan L. Regnier and the St. Paul Area YMCA
Cover design: Anne Brownfield
Text design: Mary Foster and Anne Brownfield
Compositor: Gloria Otremba
Keyliner: Don Nicholes
Interior and Cover Photographs: Thoen Photography
Illustrations: Bob Doig

Special thanks to Dan Baker, Melody Johnson, Noell Whitman, Pamela Barnard, Carol Nadlonek, Virginia Selle, Nancy Lauritsen-Smith, Sharon Stanton, Christine Larsen, Dee Marks, Katy Cooper, Andrea Sherek, and Lady Madonna Maternity Boutiques. This book would not have been possible without the cooperation and enthusiasm of our models: Carolyn Barnes; Kristin Henning and Matthew Bartel; Coral and Derek Bonin; Robert and Lindsay Collins; Cheryl Cooper; Debbie and Matthew Duncan; Joyce Miyamoto and Carly Faber; Lori Jane Hadaway; Marchelle Hallman; Pat McCarty; Linda Moskalik; Carol Nadlonek; Donna Rogers; Richard and Nickolas Rud; Cyndia and Kevin Schweiger; Susan and Diane Sherek; Peg and Meghan Short; Debbie and Benjamin Willett; and Nancy, Larry, and Nicholas Wood.

The contents of this book have been reviewed and checked for accuracy and appropriateness by medical doctors. However, the authors, editors, and publisher disclaim all responsibility arising from any adverse effects or results that occur or might occur as a result of the inappropriate application of any of the information in this book. If you have a question about the appropriateness of any exercises or treatments described in this book, consult your medical caregiver.

Contents

Dedication

I dedicate this book to women everywhere who have the common goal of staying fit during pregnancy, and who realize the necessity of getting back into shape after delivery and raising the healthiest babies possible.

To my family: husband Steve, and sons Ryan and Reid, whose love and support I feel always. We share an interest in fitness throughout life and a family bond that brings special meaning to my life.

To Beth, Susan, Ellen, Terre, and Colleen for sharing their knowledge, programs, and personal experiences to make this a truly special book. It has been a dream of mine for two years to bring together women who also were working on prenatal, postnatal, and baby fitness in the YMCAs, and who believe as strongly as I do in wellness as a way of life to be shared as a family.

Acknowledgments

This book is based on my original book, which included a foreword by Sandra Sackett, M.D.; an introduction by Rosalie Dauffenbach, R.N.; illustrations by John Boyer; and editing by Paul Kringle.

Special thanks to the members of the YMCA task force that helped me expand the You & Me, Baby program: Beth Dannhauser, Huntington, New York YMCA; Ellen Feeney-Pelliter, Eugene, Oregon YMCA; Colleen Kirby, Oklahoma City, Oklahoma YMCA; Terre Klipsch, Naperville, Illinois YMCA; Susan MacPhee, Portland, Maine YMCA; and Dr. Bill Zuti, YMCA of USA. Each of these capable people represents dozens of others who have been involved in classes on this subject.

One final acknowledgment must be made of the contributions of Tom Grady and Donna Ahrens of Meadowbrook. Their commitment to the topic has made it possible to spread the message far beyond the YMCA.

Introduction

You & Me, Baby is a book for any woman who is concerned about her own health and that of her baby. The exercise routines in the book were developed for use in YMCA fitness classes that are offered in hundreds of communities in the United States. These classes are for women who want to stay fit during pregnancy or get back into shape after delivery, and for parents of newborns who want to start their babies off on the road to fitness as a way of life.

Meadowbrook Books is making this book available to thousands of pregnant women who may not know about the YMCA classes or who would prefer to do the exercise routines on their own. Whether you obtain this book from the YMCA, a bookstore, from a friend or through a clinic or hospital program, please check with your medical caregiver to be sure he or she agrees with the information and suggestions presented here. There are many special circumstances that could influence what you should do before, during, or after your baby's birth.

You & Me, Baby is based on the original work of Susan L. Regnier, which she self-published and, more importantly, shared by training staff and volunteer leaders in local YMCAs across the country. Susan first developed the exercise routines for her own use during her first pregnancy, then taught others in the St. Paul Area YMCAs in Minnesota. In 1983, she brought together a task force of YMCA leaders who had each developed programs for their communities, to expand the program and make it a national Y effort. This process has resulted in a practical program that has been developed and tested for three years. The program has made a difference to literally thousands of women, whose participation and feedback to local YMCA staff have contributed to this book.

The contents of this book have been reviewed by Dr. Sandra Sackett, American Academy of Pediatrics and Twin City Obstetrics and Gynecology, LTD; and by Drs. John Brown, Jerome Scherek, John Farr and Robert Braun. Still, there is no substitute for a thorough discussion between you and your doctor. Share this book with your doctor and ask specifically if she or he supports your engaging in the exercise routines suggested.

You & Me, Baby is organized into four chapters. The first chapter discusses the changing human relationships in your life over the next nine months, principles of good nutrition during pregnancy, and basic physiological changes that occur during pregnancy. The chapter concludes with a detailed exercise routine that has been designed for and widely used by pregnant women across the country.

Chapter two provides a set of exercises that can help you prepare for a cesarean delivery (many such deliveries are unexpected), and exercise routines for you to use in the hospital after delivery. Whether your delivery is vaginal or cesarean, the goal is still the same—a healthy baby.

Chapter three takes up the issues of the postpartum period, including adjustments in family relationships and physical changes, and concludes with an effective exercise routine for getting back into shape.

The fourth chapter focuses on your new baby. It introduces principles of massage and provides three different types of exercise routines: one for babies from birth to four months old, another for babies from four to twelve months old, and a third that will provide exercise for both you and your baby (including a few exercises that involve *both* parents as well as the baby).

This chapter also includes practical sewing patterns to use to make your own equipment for exercise.

In the appendix you will find a list of resources—books, periodicals, and organizations—you can turn to for more information on specific topics. The appendix also includes a pregnancy primer that you may find helpful as various physiological problems and concerns arise. Again, this is not medical advice, but basic information to help you understand possible causes and treatments. It is most important to see your doctor regularly throughout your pregnancy.

The You & Me, Baby program represents "wellness" in the most fundamental sense. The wellness concept suggests that:

- Each of us is responsible for our own health.
- Our health is a gift that we must work to maintain.
- To be well involves the whole person—body, mind and spirit.
- We all need a support group—friends or relatives who care about how we feel and for whom we care in return.
- The quest for the full life is an ongoing, never-ending journey that brings both challenges and rewards every day!

The YMCA leadership and developers of the You & Me, Baby program wish you the greatest success in your journey.

Jerry Glashagel
Director of Program Development
YMCA of the USA

Chapter One
Prenatal Concerns and Exercise Routine

The benefits of exercising during pregnancy are now widely accepted by medical and fitness specialists. Many prenatal caregivers prescribe exercise, in addition to the usual vitamins, in their prenatal care instructions. Firmer, better-toned muscles help you feel better, give you added strength in areas of your body stressed by pregnancy (particularly the back, abdomen, and pelvic area), and can make your delivery and postpartum recovery easier. Evidence in studies done by the Melpomene Institute of St. Paul, Minnesota, indicates that women who exercise when they are pregnant regain their shape sooner after pregnancy than women who do not.

The prenatal exercise routine on pages 18 to 63 is designed to keep you flexible and give you control over the degrees of strength and relaxation you need during delivery. As your baby grows, the difficulty of doing the exercises will increase. If the exercise routine doesn't seem strenuous at first, be patient and think of your priorities. This routine will maintain your strength, muscle tone, and flexibility while assuring your baby's overall well-being.

There are several ways to go about your regular exercise routine. Exercising by yourself at home offers the advantages of privacy and a flexible time schedule. On the other hand, you may prefer the opportunities for support and sharing of concerns that a group exercise class with other pregnant women can provide. An exercise class at the YMCA or another fitness center provides not only the advantage of mutual encouragement, but also the leadership of a trained person who will guide you through a routine of safe exercises and can help you find the answers to questions or concerns you may have.

Exercise can be done "on land"—indoors or outdoors—or in water, which is an ideal medium for exercise, especially for pregnant women. The buoyancy of your body in water promotes flexibility and allows you to move through a wide range of motions without danger of falling. Also, the resistance property of water demands a muscular effort, which serves as an effective toner for many parts of the body (e.g., arms and legs). The same property may also help prevent injuries since potentially harmful quick, jerky motions are less likely to occur in water.

The support of the water becomes increasingly helpful as you gain extra weight in the later months of your pregnancy. Exercise remains comfortable in the water when it might not on land, especially for exercises that involve the weight-bearing joints, such as the hips, knees, and ankles. Water exercise also helps control your body temperature and aids you in relaxing and cooling down. Many women find the YMCA swimming pools and water exercise programs ideal for their workouts during pregnancy. The Y is also a great place to join a prenatal exercise class "on land," in the gym or exercise area. Most Y prenatal exercise programs use the routine at the end of this chapter.

The rest of this introduction deals with human relations during pregnancy; nutritional needs of pregnant women; physiological changes (including changes in posture) that occur during pregnancy; and the cardiovascular system and its importance in preparing for labor and delivery. The chapter concludes with a description of basic exercise positions, breathing techniques, and the prenatal exercise routine.

Human Relations

Having a baby involves not just yourself, but a group of people—your partner, parents, grandparents, friends, perhaps other children, a doctor or midwife, and other members of the medical community. Each of these people affects how you feel. Your concerns about your own health and the health of your baby will be influenced by their reactions to your pregnancy and by the advice they offer you.

What you do about your health and fitness will, in turn, affect the lives of others. Exercise routines and eating habits, for example, are not strictly individual matters. Meals are generally important times for communicating as a family, and exercise and leisure activities often involve the whole family. How you get along with your partner, your friends, your relatives, and the new members of your private world from the medical community will make a difference in your social and mental health. During pregnancy, your attitude, which is highly influenced by your relationships with others, is a crucial component of your overall fitness.

The importance of developing and maintaining good relationships cannot be overemphasized. The three basic elements of good human relations are self-esteem, communication, and trust. During pregnancy, taking care of your mental health—by knowing what will make you feel good about yourself and by seeking those things out—is crucial to your self-esteem. In addition, your relationships with your medical caregivers, your husband, and others will benefit if you speak frankly about what you are thinking and feeling, and ask them to do the same. Finally, by respecting the

rights of others to express themselves freely, you will help foster the mutual trust and respect that are vital to good communication and self-esteem.

Nutrition

Pregnancy is not the time to try the latest fad diets. Rather, it is a time to learn about and use principles of sound nutrition, since what you consume will affect both you and your baby. Learn as much about nutrition as you can so that you can plan what you eat. You needn't draw up menus to cover long periods of time—just keep in mind what you have on hand, how much time you have, and so on, to help you produce healthy, balanced meals. This may take some effort at first, but in time it will become second nature.

The major principle of good nutrition can be easily summed up: eat enough of what you need and not too much of what you don't need. But identifying what you do and don't need can be tricky, and applying that knowledge may be harder still. Fortunately, foods can be combined in an infinite number of ways to produce a healthful diet.

What does your body need? Food and water. More specifically, your body needs about fifty nutrients that it cannot manufacture for itself. Basically, these nutrients are proteins, vitamins, and minerals. Because no one food has all the nutrients you need, you should eat some of each of the four basic food types—protein suppliers, fruits and vegetables, grains, and milk and milk products—every day. Some foods fit into two categories—for example, milk and some legumes and grains are also good protein sources, and meat is a good source of iron, a mineral.

Protein Suppliers

Protein is made up of amino acids. Your body needs eight amino acids that it cannot produce itself.

Complete protein is available from animal products— meat, fish, poultry, eggs, and milk. Grains, legumes (peas, beans, nuts), and seeds provide protein, but no grain, legume, or seed alone provides a complete protein. However, they can be mixed or combined with milk or cheese to provide protein as complete as that available in animal products. For example, peanut butter on whole wheat bread, beans and rice, and oatmeal and milk work complimentarily to produce complete protein.

Fruits and Vegetables

Fruits and vegetables provide minerals and vitamins, carbohydrates for your body to burn, and fiber for better digestion. Processing and preparation affect the nutritional value of these foods; for example, heat causes some vitamins, particularly vitamin C, to break down. Fresh, raw vegetables provide the most nutrition; other forms of preparation provide less. The blanching and heat sealing involved in the commercial canning of vegetables can significantly decrease their nutritional worth.

Cereals

Cereals include whole and enriched grains, rice, bread, noodles, and spaghetti. They supply protein, carbohydrates, fiber, vitamins, and minerals.

Milk and Milk Products

This food group includes milk, cheese, yogurt, and cottage cheese. Milk and milk products are good sources of calcium, vitamin D, and protein.

Special Issues

Within the context of the principles of sound nutrition are several special issues related to pregnancy. One of these issues has to do with how much you eat. A common problem in the first three months of pregnancy is lack of appetite, often accompanied by vomiting. This is the time to talk with your caregiver about food supplements or vitamins. He or she may suggest supplements to make up for nutrients not eaten or lost through vomiting. You may also need to compensate for an overall lack of calories.

Do not take food supplements or vitamins during your pregnancy without first checking with your doctor.

Basic Food Group Servings

The Proteins Group

Recommended minimum during pregnancy: Three to four servings per day.

What is a serving?

1 small chicken leg
1/2 small chicken breast
2 slices of chicken, turkey, veal, lamb, liver, beef, ham, or pork
1 hamburger patty
2 eggs
1/2 cup cottage cheese
2 slices of cheddar cheese
1 cup cooked beans or lentils, combined with rice, macaroni, or bread
4 T. peanut butter and one slice of bread

The Fruits and Vegetables Group

Recommended minimum during pregnancy: Four servings per day.

What is a serving?

1 cup raw salad (excluding dressing)
1/2 cup cooked fruit or vegetables
1 medium cantaloupe
1/2 cup berries
10-12 grapes or cherries
1/2 medium banana or grapefruit
2 medium plums, nectarines
1 medium pear, orange, apple
6 oz. unsweetened fruit juice

The Breads and Cereals Group

Recommended minimum during pregnancy: Four servings per day.

What is a serving?

1 slice of bread
1/2 - 3/4 cup cooked cereal
1 roll, biscuit or muffin
1 oz. (about 1 cup) ready-to-eat cereal
1/2 - 3/4 cup cooked macaroni, spaghetti, or noodles

The Milk Group

Recommended minimum during pregnancy: Four servings per day.

What is a serving?

1 cup milk
1 slice of Swiss cheese
1 cup yogurt
1 cup custard
1 cup cottage cheese

Typical Weight Gain Distribution During Pregnancy	
Placenta	1.4 lbs.
Uterus	2.0 lbs.
Blood	4.0 lbs.
Baby	7.7 lbs.
Amniotic Fluid	1.8 lbs.
Breast Tissue	0.9 lbs.
Tissue Fluid	2.7 lbs.
Other	3.5 lbs.
TOTAL	24.0 lbs.

Excessive amounts of some vitamins, such as A and D, can harm your baby. On the other hand, all of your nutrient needs are greater during pregnancy, and the need for iron is nearly impossible to meet without a supplement. Your caregiver may recommend supplements to increase your intake of iron and other vitamins and minerals.

The issue of how much weight you can expect to gain safely with appropriate eating should be answered by your doctor. The chart at left lists some of the common weight-gain categories for a woman who gained twenty-four pounds on the way to delivering a seven-pound, seven-ounce baby.

Other Health Concerns

There are several other *don'ts* related to substances that can be particularly dangerous to good health during pregnancy:

• *Don't smoke.* Current research suggests that smoking during pregnancy is associated with low birth weight and with an increase of miscarriages and stillbirths. You should also avoid contact with smokers as much as possible, since there is increasing evidence that sidestream smoke is unhealthy for those who inhale it. In fact, the people who breathe in the smoke from another person's cigarette can ingest more of several harmful smoke by-products than the smoker does.

• *Don't drink alcoholic beverages.* In a number of ways, alcohol can pose a threat to the unborn baby. Alcohol can interfere with the normal growth process of fetal cells. The percentage of alcohol in the bloodstream of the developing baby is the same as the percentage of alcohol in the mother's bloodstream.

• *Cut down on or eliminate caffeine.* The caffeine in coffee, tea, cola drinks, chocolate, and many over-the-counter medications stimulates the central nervous system. The use of caffeine can be related to nervousness, restlessness, insomnia, and heartburn. Current research is also investigating the possible relationship between consumption of large amounts of caffeine and birth defects. The safe thing to do is to cut out caffeine altogether during pregnancy.

• *Don't take any medication or drug without first discussing it with your doctor.* Aspirin, antihistamines, sleeping aids, and, for some people, marijuana and other drugs have become part of everyday life. Because these substances can influence the early development of the baby, it is advisable to discontinue use of all medications and drugs, especially during the first three months of pregnancy. If you feel you need any medication, talk to your doctor to see what he or she recommends.

Conclusion

Pregnancy is a time to eat a balanced diet of healthy foods and to feel good as a result. A feeling of vitality comes from eating just enough of a variety of foods from the four basic groups. Feeling good never comes from overeating, or from consuming large quantities of fats and of high-calorie goodies. Your pregnancy is a perfect time to explore truly good eating habits and to discover the pleasures of feeling really good when you eat correctly!

Pregnancy Primer

The pregnancy primer on pages 180 to 182 lists fourteen problems commonly associated with pregnancy (e.g., nausea, varicose veins, stretch marks), together with possible causes and solutions. However, this information should by no means be considered a substitute for a discussion with your medical caregiver about any physiological or psychological concerns you have during your pregnancy.

Physiology

A number of changes occur in your body during pregnancy; there are new feelings and, sometimes, discomforts to contend with. And the final act of labor is plain hard work. You will find each stage of pregnancy more manageable if you understand what is going on in your body and if you work to keep your muscles and your entire cardiovascular system in the best possible condition.

Several major changes in your physiology occur during pregnancy:

• Your uterus increases in size to accommodate the growing baby. As it stretches it may cause some discomfort in your internal ligament support structures.

• Your uterus, which is located in the pelvic cavity bordered in back by the spinal column, is pushed forward into the abdominal wall as it increases in size.

• Your vagina and birth canal are supported by the pelvic floor musculature. As your uterus enlarges, your vagina is subjected to pressure.

• Your gastrointestinal system can be upset as a result of pressure on and displacement of your stomach and intestines as your uterus enlarges.

• Your breasts usually increase in size and become tender.

• Your blood volume can increase by 30 to 50 percent, and your heart rate may increase an average of ten to fifteen beats per minute. Generally blood pressure does not increase despite the increase in blood volume and heart rate.

• Your respiratory system is affected in two ways. Your lung capacity may be reduced as your uterus enlarges and your diaphragm moves up. Also, hormones released during pregnancy can cause your body to be more sensitive to carbon dioxide, resulting in an increased likelihood of rapid fatigue from vigorous activity.

There is little, if anything, you can do to prevent breast tenderness or discomfort caused by the stretching of the ligaments of your uterus. However, you can reduce some of the other major physiological discomforts by doing specific exercises to strengthen your pelvic floor and abdominal muscles, and by performing regular exercise to keep your cardiovascular system in good shape. These exercises and cardiovascular concerns are discussed in the following pages.

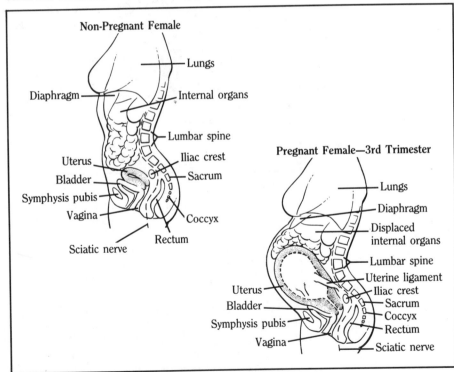

Pelvic Floor Musculature and the Kegel Exercise

In preparing for delivery, it is important that you understand the pelvic floor musculature and practice the "kegel" exercise, which involves contracting your pelvic floor muscles. The exercise was named for Dr. Arnold Kegel, one of the first physicians to stress the importance of the pelvic floor musculature.

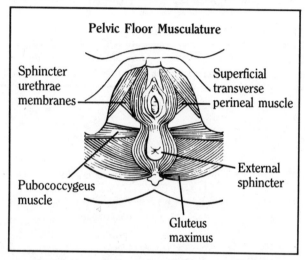

Pelvic Floor Musculature

Sphincter urethrae membranes

Superficial transverse perineal muscle

Pubococcygeus muscle

External sphincter

Gluteus maximus

The hammocklike pelvic floor (or perineal) muscles, which stretch from your pubic bone to your tailbone (coccyx), support your pelvic organs such as the uterus, bladder, and bowel. Your pelvic floor also relaxes and contracts when you urinate. During pregnancy, your pelvic floor muscles may sag in response to hormonal changes and the increasing weight of your uterus.

Because the condition of the pelvic floor muscles is of lifelong importance, doing the kegel exercise regularly is essential both during pregnancy and throughout your lifetime. Among the many benefits of maintaining the muscle tone of your pelvic floor are increased sup-

port of your pelvic organs and better bladder control. Long-term benefits include proper positioning of your internal organs within your pelvic area.

To become aware of the muscles you are exercising when you "kegel," try to stop the flow of urine as you urinate. (You may practice in this fashion while you are learning to kegel, but you should not use this method continuously.)

The kegel exercise can be done in any position. Think of the pelvic floor as an elevator. Contract your pelvic floor muscles a little at a time, as if you are going up the floors from ground to fifth floor. Hold the muscles tightly at the top, then slowly release them as you descend to the ground floor. When you arrive at the ground floor, think "release" to try to relax the muscles even further. This should be done smoothly and gradually. Do not hold your breath while you are doing the kegel exercise.

Kegels can be done during intercourse with your partner, who can give you feedback on how you are doing. As an added bonus, your kegels may enhance your partner's sexual response. You should start doing kegels now, do them throughout your pregnancy, do a kegel or relax your pelvic floor during labor and pushing, and continue to do kegels after delivery to promote healing of your perineum and to restore your pelvic floor to its original tone and keep it that way.

Recti Diastasis

During pregnancy, you may experience some degree of recti diastasis, or separation of the abdominal muscles. Especially in the second trimester of pregnancy, your abdominal (rectus) muscles are susceptible to the internal pressure exerted by your uterus as the baby pushes from within it. The structure of the female abdominal muscles make it possible for them to separate at the center seam (linea alba) that runs vertically down the middle of your abdomen.

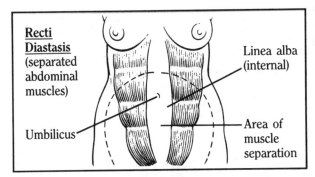

Recti Diastasis (separated abdominal muscles)

Linea alba (internal)

Umbilicus

Area of muscle separation

Separation of the abdominal muscles is caused by a combination of hormonal changes, excessive strain, and sudden jerking movements. It is important that you regain the stability and integrity of separated abdominal muscles by performing specific abdominal exercises as soon as possible after delivery.

The exercises in this book are intended to help you maintain and regain the strength and tone of your abdominal muscles. However, before beginning any of the exercise routines, have your doctor check for abdominal muscle separation, or use the self-test below.

1. Lie on your back with your knees bent, your heels by your hips.
2. Place your fingertips on your abdomen, on the soft tissue area just above your navel. Use your navel as a "landmark" to keep your fingertips in place.
3. Pull your chin to your chest and curl your shoulders off the floor while pressing firmly on your abdomen with your fingers.
4. Feel for the tautness of the muscle bands and gauge the size of the soft region between these bands. Any width greater than approximately one inch should be treated with caution, and indicates that you should progress gradually in the degree of difficulty for the abdominal exercises in this book.

Posture

Another important physiologic concern during pregnancy is posture. Your posture will change dramatically and quickly as your uterus enlarges and your abdominal muscles are stretched to capacity. The strain is felt on your distended abdomen and in the increased lumbar (low back) spinal curve. Your spine, particularly in the lumbar region, becomes an anchor that compensates for the gradual shift in your center of gravity. As the abdominal distension and spinal curvature increase, you may begin to lean back on your heels, thereby further increasing the lumbar curve. This "swaybacked" posture will, in turn, tend to increase the likelihood and severity of lower back pain.

Poor posture is generally caused by a lack of integrity of the abdominal and gluteal (buttock) muscles. When your abdominal and gluteal muscles are working together to keep your pelvis positioned properly, your spine can keep your head and shoulders in proper alignment. If your gluteal muscles are tight, your quadriceps (thigh muscles) will relax, which in turn will keep your knees from hyperextending. Your feet will then be

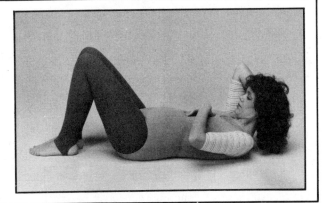

Self-Test for Separation of the Abdominal Muscles (Recti Diastasis)

better able to support your added body weight without being forced to point outward in the so-called "pregnant waddle."

Your pelvis, which supports your spinal column, takes on an important role in your posture during pregnancy. The increasing weight of your uterus and stretching of your uterine wall will cause your pelvis to tend to angle forward. Therefore, it is especially important during pregnancy that you keep your pelvis tilted back in order to maintain good posture and minimize lumbar curve. Performing the Tuck and Pull exercise (below), which involves "tucking" your pelvis in and pulling in your abdominal muscles, will help you do so.

Tuck and Pull Exercise

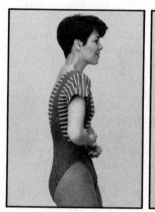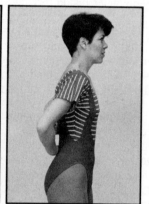

Practicing this exercise whenever possible will help promote good posture during pregnancy. The movements you perform in doing the exercise precede many specific prenatal and postnatal exercises. Learn to move smoothly through the exercise so that the individual actions "flow" as a natural movement.

In this exercise, the muscles of your trunk work together to perform the pelvic tilt (tuck):

1. Stand with your knees unlocked and slightly bent. "Tuck" your pelvis in and pull in your abdominal muscles (this allows for a pelvic rocking action).
2. Contract your secondary abdominal muscles and buttocks (this allows your diaphragm to expand and flattens your lower back).

The Cardiovascular System

Because the maternal circulatory system is the source of fetal oxygen and nutrition, the condition of your heart and lung (cardiovascular) system during pregnancy makes a difference in the amount of oxygen-rich blood your baby will receive. The condition of this system will improve with regular exercise. If you have been exercising regularly, being pregnant is no reason to quit. On the contrary, it is a good reason to continue. If you have not been working out, now is the time to start!

An important component of the cardiovascular portion of the workout is monitoring your target heart rate. Your target heart rate is the rate at which your heart ideally should be beating during the part of the workout—walking or jogging, for example—when your body demands, produces, and distributes more oxygen than usual over a sustained period of time (generally, twenty to thirty minutes).

The target heart rate training zone chart on page 9 shows the normal target-heart-rate range by age, and a special pregnancy target-heart-rate range (also by age), which is slightly below the normal target range. It is important to work up to the level of the lower number, but not higher than the higher number, and to sustain that workload for twenty to thirty minutes.

Recommended Training Zone for Prenatal Women, by Heart Rate and Age

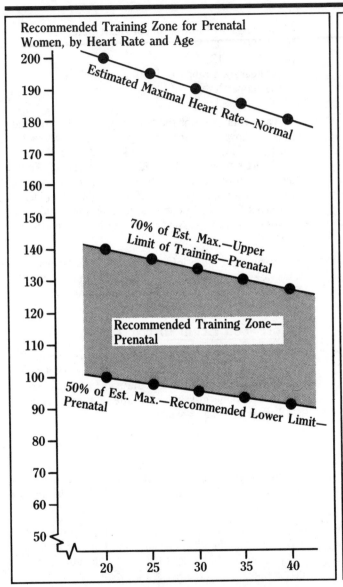

Estimated Maximal Heart Rate—Normal

70% of Est. Max.—Upper Limit of Training—Prenatal

Recommended Training Zone—Prenatal

50% of Est. Max.—Recommended Lower Limit—Prenatal

Predicted Maximal 70% and 50% Heart Rate by Age

Age	Predicted Max	70% (10 sec.)	50% (10 sec.)
20	200	140	100
21	199	139	
22	198	139	99
23	197	138	
24	196	138	98
25	195	137	
26	194	136	97
27	193	135	
28	192	134	96
29	191	134	
30	190	133	95
31	189	132	
32	188	131	94
33	187	131	
34	186	130	93
35	185	129	
36	184	128	92
37	183	128	
38	182	127	91
39	181	126	
40	180	126	90
41	179	125	
42	178	125	89
43	177	124	
44	176	123	88
45	175	123	

Conversion of Heart Rate (bpm) to 10 Second Count

Maximal Heart Rate	70% (10 sec.)	50% (10 sec.)	Age
200	23		20
199	"		21
198	"		22
197	"		23
196	"		24
195	"		25
194	"		26
193	"		27
192	22	16	28
191	"		29
190	"		30
189	"		31
188	"		32
187	"		33
186	"		34
185	"		35
184	21		36
183	"		37
182	"		38
181	"		39
180	"	15	40
179	"		41
178	"		42
177	"		43
176	"		44
175	20		45

Source: Astrand, modification based on 220 - Age = Max HR

To determine your target heart rate:

1. Press the fingertips of your right hand firmly into your left wrist, just below your left thumb. *Do not* use your thumb to take your pulse; it has a pulse of its own.

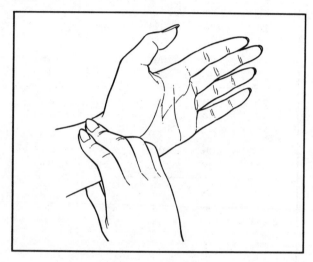

2. Take your pulse, using a watch or clock with a second hand as you count the beats.

3. Count the pulse beats for ten seconds and multiply by six for a minute count; or take a six-second count and multiply by ten.

4. Use the target heart rate chart to find your ideal target-heart-rate range.

5. If you choose not to use the chart, you can use the following formula: Take your age and subtract it from 220 to find your maximum heart rate. Your target-heart-rate range is fifty to seventy percent of your maximum heart rate. *Example:* If you are 30 years old, calculate your target-heart-rate range as follows:

220-30 (age) = 190 (Maximum Heart Rate)
.50 × 190 = 95
.70 × 190 = 133
Target-heart-rate range = 95 (lower level) to
    133 (upper level)

Take your pulse at the beginning, middle, and end of the cardiovascular portion of your exercise workout—e.g., before and after walking or jogging—and check your heart rate at the very end of your workout. Your pulse should be between sixteen and eighteen beats, or lower, in a ten-second count. If it is higher than eighteen beats, be sure to continue to cool down until you are within this range. Never work up to your maximum heart rate.

If you want more information about target heart rates, ask the trained fitness leaders at your local YMCA or another physical fitness organization.

Before You Begin to Exercise

Remember that many prenatal exercises can be done in water as well as on land. In the prenatal exercise routine (pages 18 to 63), the name of any exercise that can be done in water with little or no modification is followed by a water symbol:

Before you begin the prenatal exercise routine, you'll want to review these general principles of sound exercise programs:

• Check with your doctor before starting an exercise program. You should be healthy and have no complicating medical problems before starting such a program. Look over the exercises in this book, then consult your doctor to make sure there are no reasons why you should not do any of them.

• Check for separation of your abdominal muscles, using the self-test on page 7, or have your doctor check to see whether you should take care in doing (or avoid doing) any of the exercises designed to strengthen and maintain the tone of your abdominal muscles.

• During the first three months of pregnancy, monitor your body temperature when exercising. It is important that you not raise the core body temperature above 100 degrees F. during this period, since the developing baby does not yet have the ability to dissipate body heat. Thus, avoid overexercising in a hot environment or otherwise raising your body temperature.

• Begin your exercise routine slowly, taking care to do the warm-up exercises first. Do easy stretching and loosening-up exercises before engaging in cardiovascular exercise.

• If a position in any exercise is uncomfortable, adjust to a similar position that feels more comfortable.

• The suggested number of repetitions for each exercise is only a recommendation; you may want to do fewer or more than the number specified, depending on your fitness level.

• If you feel a strain or pain of any kind, stop exercising and rest for a few moments. The next time you try that exercise, remember to take it easy.

• To get the maximum benefit from the exercise routine, do as much of each exercise as possible, do as many exercises in the routine as you can, and follow the order in which the exercises are given.

• Follow exercising with a cool-down period. A simple cool-down routine will help you begin to relax, get your heart rate back to normal, and allow your muscles to comfortably return to their unstretched state.

• Take your pulse at the beginning, middle, and end of the cardiovascular portion of the routine. Then check your recovery heart rate at the very end of your workout. (For information on target heart rate, see pages 8 to 10.)

Using This Book at Home

If you are using this book on your own, rather than in conjunction with a You & Me, Baby exercise class, you'll benefit most from the prenatal exercise routine if you perform it at least three times a week. The exercises are intended to be performed in the order in which they are presented here. Be sure to read the instructions above in "Before you Begin to Exercise" before beginning the exercise routine.

Sitting Positions

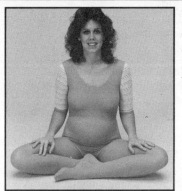

Tailor Sit
Sit tall, with your spine erect, and fold your legs comfortably in front of your body.

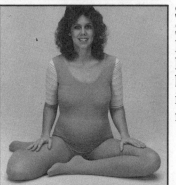

Side Sit
Sit tall, with both your knees bent, so that your left ankle is close to your body and your right ankle is away from your body (or reverse the leg positions).

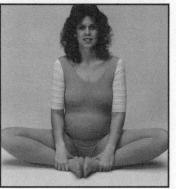

Butterfly Sit
Sit tall, with your spine erect and the soles of your feet touching.

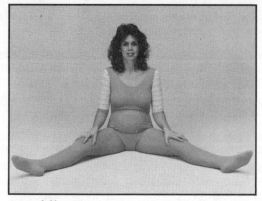

Straddle Sit
Sit tall, with your spine erect, and extend your legs in front of your body in a V position.

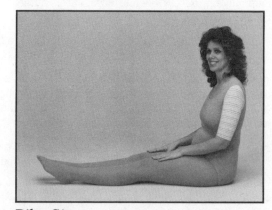

Pike Sit
Sit tall, with your spine erect, and extend your legs directly in front of your body, so that your body forms an L.

Arm Positions

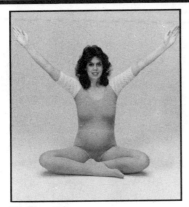

V Position
Extend your arms
overhead in a V.

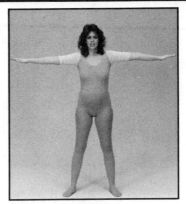

Cross Position
Extend your arms out to
your sides at shoulder
level.

Feet Positions

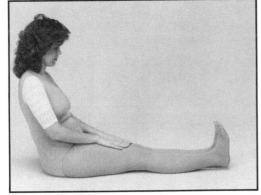

Feet Flexed
Sit tall, holding your spine erect.
Extend your legs in front of you
with your feet perpendicular to the
floor and toes pointed up.

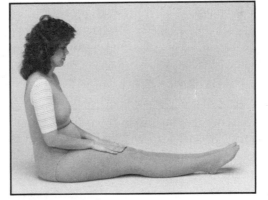

Toes Pointed
Sit tall, holding your spine erect.
Extend your legs in front of you,
pointing your toes straight out from
your body.

13

Body Positions

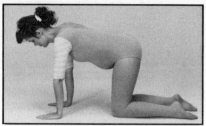

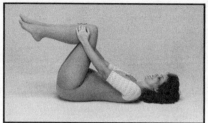

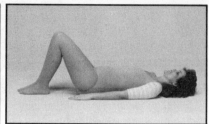

All Fours
Roll over to your hands and knees. Strive to keep your body balanced so that your shoulders are aligned with your flat palms and your hips are aligned with your knees.

Back Tuck
Lie flat on your back and draw both knees into your chest or around your belly. Keep your back flat on the floor.

Hook-Lying
Lie flat on your back with your knees bent and your feet flat on the floor.

Rolling to a Standing Position

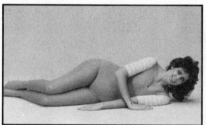

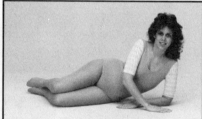

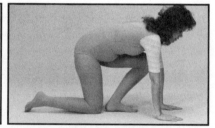

Whenever you move from a lying position to a standing position when you are pregnant, begin by rolling onto your side.

Place the palm of your hand flat on the floor to gently raise your upper body, then gradually roll to your knees. Once you are on all fours, place your feet flat on the floor, one at a time.

To straighten up from a forward-leaning position (i.e., upper body hanging loosely), bend your knees so that your thigh muscles can assist in lifting your upper body weight. When your upper body is straight, straighten your knees to stand.

Because proper breathing helps you to relax and relieves tension, it can help during labor as well as when you exercise. When you do the exercises in the prenatal and post-partum routines, inhale as you relax and exhale as you hold a stretch or isometric contraction.

The following breathing exercises are most beneficial when done during a warm-up or cool-down routine, or whenever you need to relax. To do the exercises properly, keep your spine straight and your eyes open, and clear your mind of everything but your breathing. Breathe slowly, quietly, and continuously, taking air in through your nose to purify it. Work up gradually to a comfortable limit of air; taking in too much air can cause over-oxidation and hyperventilation or dizziness.

Aim: To teach you to breathe down into your diaphragm.

Starting Position: Tailor sit, with your hands on your stomach and the fingertips of your middle fingers touching lightly.

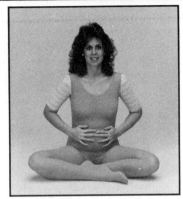

Simple Breath

1 Breathing in through your nose, bring air into your lungs and allow it to push your stomach outward. Your fingertips should move apart slightly as your stomach expands. Hold your breath for a count of five, then slowly exhale (this will bring your fingertips back together). *Repetitions:* Repeat slowly three to four times.

Aim: To teach you to breathe with your body movements and to expand your rib cage, giving your heart more room to work in.

Starting Position: Straddle sit, with your arms at your sides.

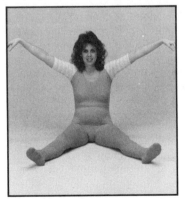

Swan Breath

1 Bring your arms into cross position, inhaling through your nose as you move your arms upward. Exhale through your mouth while bringing your arms down. *Repetitions:* Repeat three to four times.

Sniffing and Vitalic Breath

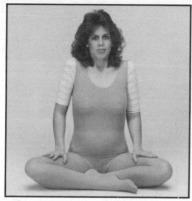

Aim: To cleanse and strengthen your lungs (many pregnant women have trouble breathing, with the symptoms of a cold, or have allergies).

Starting Position: Tailor sit.

1 Breathe a series of sharp sniffs through your nose until your lungs are completely full, then blow the air out sharply through your mouth, with a loud "HAAA." *Repetitions:* Repeat three to four times.

Alternate Nostril Breathing

Aim: To create a natural tranquilizing effect, calm your nervous system, and clear your sinuses.

Starting Position: Tailor sit.

Note: No one with high blood pressure or heart problems should hold her breath. You can, however, still benefit from this exercise by inhaling in one nostril and exhaling immediately out the other. Do not hold both nostrils closed.

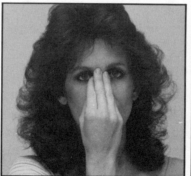

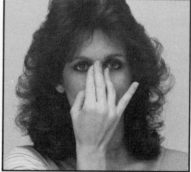

1 With the middle fingers of your right hand between your eyebrows, place your right thumb on your right nostril and your little finger on your left nostril. Relax your fingers and exhale through both nostrils.

2 Close your right nostril with your thumb and inhale in your left nostril to a count of four. Hold both nostrils closed to a count of four. Open your right nostril and exhale to a count of four. Repeat, closing your left nostril. *Repetitions:* Repeat the entire sequence three to four times.

Invigorating Breath

Aim: To ease tension and relax your lower back muscles and hamstrings.

Starting Position: Standing erect.

1 Inhale deeply while extending your arms straight out in front of you, with your palms down (this action fills the lower part of your lungs).

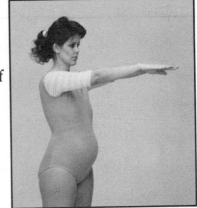

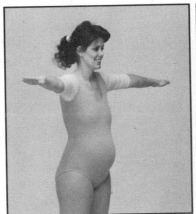

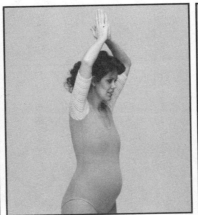

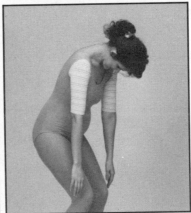

2 Inhale again and extend your arms sideways, with your palms down (this action fills the middle part of your lungs).

3 Inhale as you move your arms overhead (keeping your arms straight) until your palms touch (this action fills the upper portion of your lungs).

4 Completely relax your body. Exhale through your mouth as you let your upper body fall forward like a limp rag doll, flexing your knees slightly and keeping your fingers as close to the floor as possible.

Head Arcs

Aim: To loosen up your neck and shoulders.

Starting Position: Tailor sit.

Note: If you feel dizzy or light-headed, stop and try the exercise later or at another exercise session. *Do not* roll your head back during the exercise.

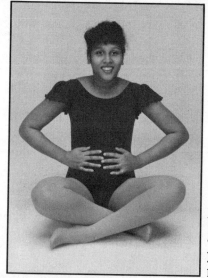

1 Begin with a few simple breaths (breathe in through your nose, bringing air into your stomach; hold your breath for a count of five, then slowly exhale).

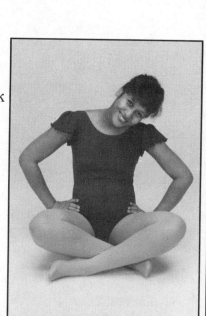

2 Drop your left ear to your left shoulder.

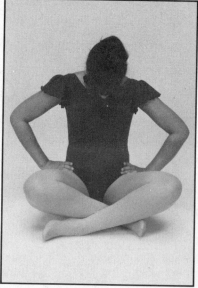

3 Gently roll your head forward to the center of your body, then drop your right ear to your right shoulder and return to starting position. *Repetitions:* Repeat three times in each direction.

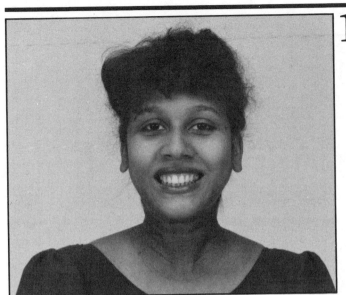

1 Smile.

⬦ Face Exercise

Aim: To tighten your facial muscles.

Starting Position: Tailor sit.

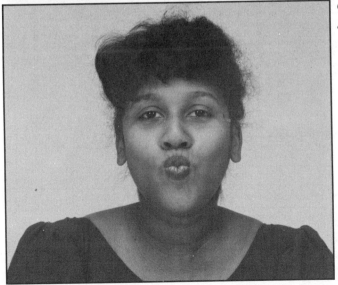

2 Pucker your face, then relax.

Exercise No. 3

Hip/Knee Rotations

Aim: To promote flexibility in your hip and knee joints.

Starting Position: Hook-lying, resting comfortably on your forearms.

To do this exercise in water, stand against the wall of the pool and raise your knees to hip level.

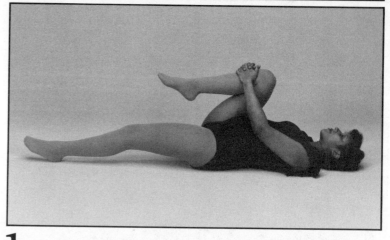

1 Raise your right knee to your chest.

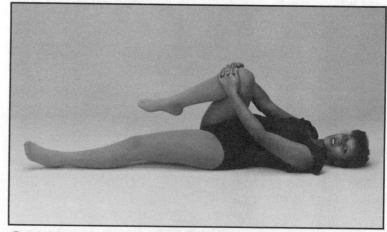

2 Holding your right knee, trace a large circle directly in front of your body with your right leg. Rotate your leg ten times to the left, then ten times to the right. *Repetitions:* Repeat with your left leg.

1 *Rotations:* Raise your shoulders to your ears. Pull your shoulders back and downward, then up and forward.

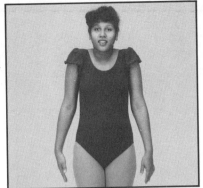

2 With your left shoulder, "draw" three circles forward, then three circles backward. Repeat with your right shoulder. Draw three circles forward with both shoulders, then reverse and draw three circles backward.

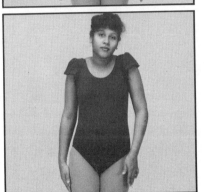

⬤ Shoulders

Aim: To loosen up your shoulders and tone your upper arms.

Starting Position: Standing with your feet slightly apart and your arms at your sides; may also be done sitting.

1 *Lifts:* Lift your shoulders and roll them forward. With your palms facing out, bring your arms forward until your little fingers touch.

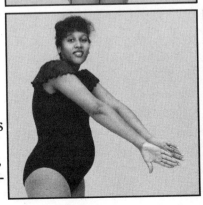

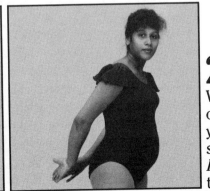

2 Lift your shoulders again and roll them backwards. With your palms still facing out, bring your arms behind your body until you feel the stretch in your shoulders. *Repetitions:* Repeat three times.

Exercise No. 4

Shoulders ◊

Aim: To loosen up your shoulders and tone your upper arms.

Starting Position: Standing with your feet slightly apart and your arms at your sides; may also be done sitting.

Note: Never drop your head and shoulders to the back.

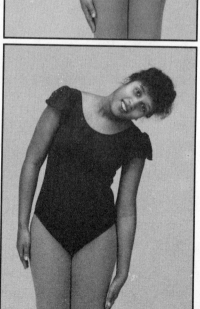

1 *Triangles:* Stabilize your abdominal region and tighten your buttocks. Move your head and your right shoulder slightly forward and to the right.

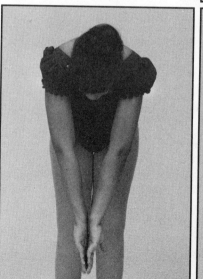

2 Roll both shoulders forward and let your head drop forward slightly.

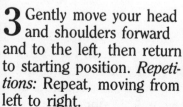

3 Gently move your head and shoulders forward and to the left, then return to starting position. *Repetitions:* Repeat, moving from left to right.

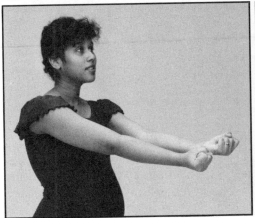

1 *Curls:* Squeeze your hands to form fists.

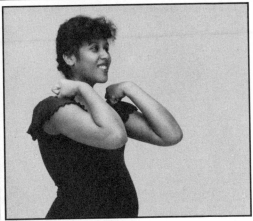

2 Touch your fists to your shoulders, then straighten your arms.
Repetitions: Repeat three to five times.

◊Arms

Aim: To tone and loosen up your arms, wrists, and fingers.

Starting Position: Standing or sitting with your arms straight out in front of you, palms up.

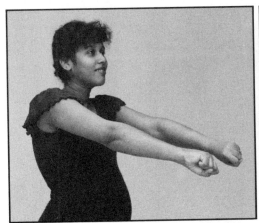

1 *Wrist Rotations:* Make fists and circle them a few times to the left, then a few times to the right.

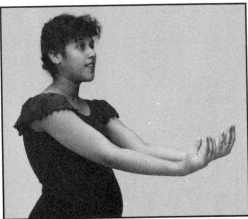

1 *Finger Flowers:* Make fists, then slowly open your fingers like a flower opening.

Exercise No. 6

Raggedy Ann

Aim: To loosen up and relax your body, particularly your neck, shoulders, and legs. This exercise can be done at any time during the exercise routine.

Starting Position: Standing with your legs slightly apart and your arms above your head.

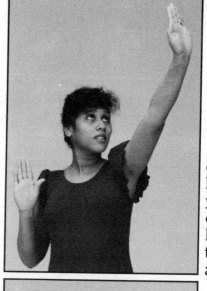

1 Press the palm of your left hand toward the ceiling, stretching the entire left side of your body until your left heel rises slightly off the floor. *Repetitions:* Repeat on your right side, then on your left side, then again on your right side.

2 With your knees slightly bent, round your shoulders and raise your arms to shoulder level. Alternately press forward with your left hand, then with your right hand, as if pushing an object away.

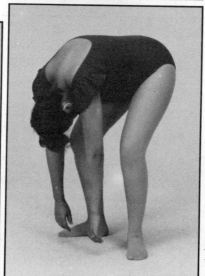

3 Keeping your hips aligned with your shoulders, drop your arms forward, drop your chin to your chest, round your shoulders forward, and bend your knees. Holding your body in a slightly flexed position, dangle for five to ten seconds. With your chin on your chest, roll up to starting position. *Repetitions:* Repeat the entire exercise one to three times.

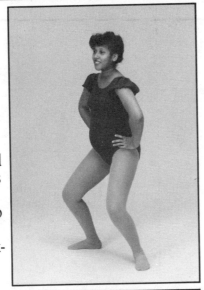

1 Slowly bend your knees outward over your feet. Go down only as far as is comfortably possible without bending forward. Strive to keep your shoulders aligned with your hips. When you have achieved maximum stretch, push your heels to the floor.

◊ Pliés

Aim: To strengthen your lower back and legs.

Starting Position: Standing erect with your feet shoulders'-width apart.

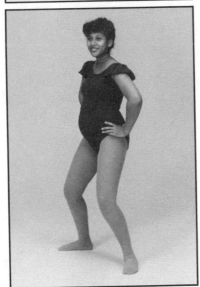

2 Press your thighs inward and slowly push your trunk upward, gradually straightening your knees. *Repetitions:* Repeat five to fifteen times.

25

Floor Sweeps

Aim: To strengthen your shoulders, lower back, and legs.

Starting Position: Standing with your legs apart with your arms in cross position.

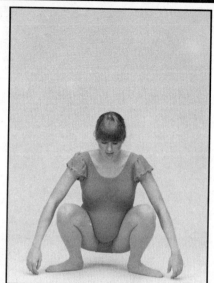

1 Bend your knees. As you bend down, swing your arms downward and cross your wrists.

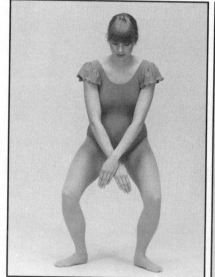

2 Begin to straighten up. As you do so, swing your arms upward and cross your wrists.

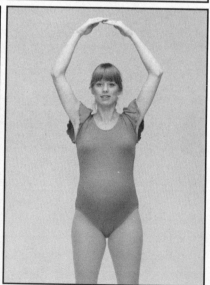

3 Complete a figure eight by crossing your hands above your head, then return to starting position. *Repetitions:* Repeat five times.

26

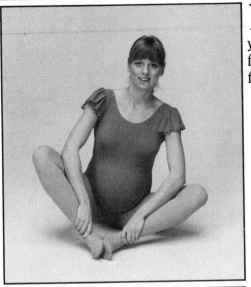

1 Place your hands on your ankles. Keeping your back straight, rock from side to side three to five times.

Butterfly Rock

Aim: To stretch your inner thighs and help prepare you for delivery.

Starting Position: Butterfly sit.

Butterfly Press

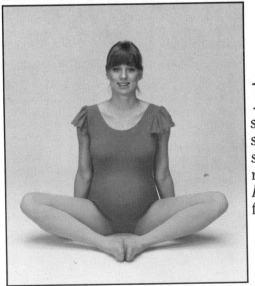

1 Put your hands on the floor by your hips for support. Keeping your back straight, press your knees slowly to the floor, then return to starting position. *Repetitions:* Repeat three to five times.

Note: As you gain flexibility, bring your feet closer toward your body for more stretching.

Exercise No. 11

Curl Ups

Aim: To strengthen your abdominal muscles and lower back.

Starting Position: Hook-lying.

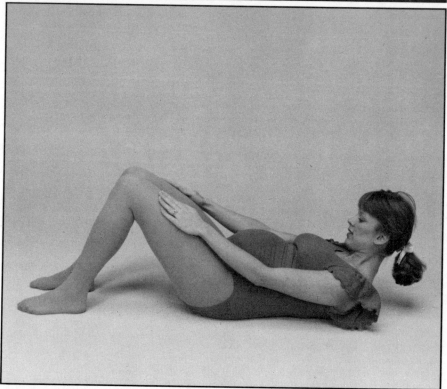

1 Holding your chin to your chest, curl up slowly just far enough for your shoulder blades to come off the floor. Hold your head and neck tightly in a fixed position for a few seconds, then lower your back to the floor. *Repetitions:* Repeat five to ten times.

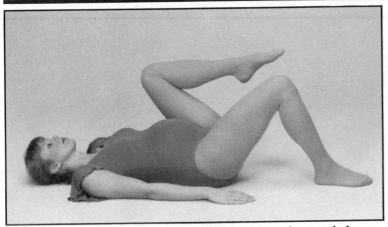

1 Draw your left leg to your chest. Extend your left leg to the ceiling, pointing your toes as you do so. Press your lower back to the floor.

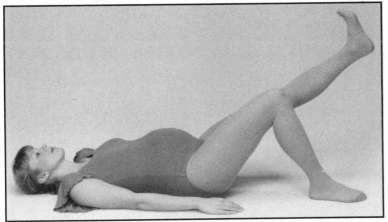

2 Flex your left foot and lower your leg slowly to the floor. *Repetitions:* Repeat three to five times with your left leg, then three to five times with your right leg.

Leg Raisers

Aim: To strengthen your abdominal and buttock muscles, lower back, and legs.

Starting Position: Hook-lying.

Pelvic Rock
(on your back)

Aim: To soothe your lower back, strengthen your abdominal muscles, and prepare you for delivery.

Starting Position: Hook-lying.

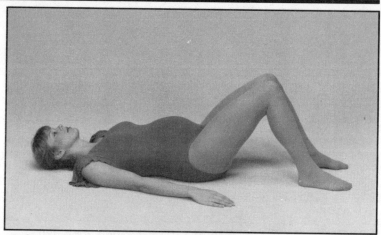

1 Press your lower back to the floor. Hold this position for a few seconds, then relax. *Repetitions:* Repeat five times *slowly*.

Raise and Roll

Aim: To strengthen your abdominal muscles, quadriceps, ankles, buttocks, and outer thigh muscles.

Starting Position: Lying on your left side with your left knee bent, resting on your shoulder with your left hand supporting your head.

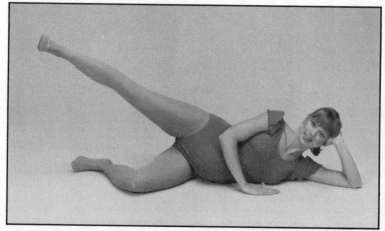

1 Raise your right leg to a comfortable height and hold it there. Circle your foot to the left, then to the right.

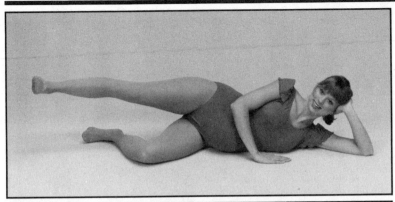

2 Lower your leg to a middle position, hold it there, and circle your foot again.

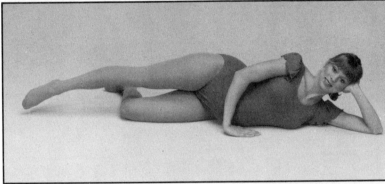

3 Lower your leg to a horizontal position and circle your foot. *Repetitions:* Repeat steps 1 through 3 three to five times.

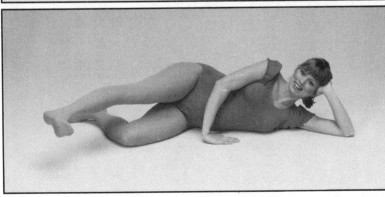

4 With your knees meeting and your left knee still bent, extend your right leg in front of you. With your foot flexed, raise your right leg hip-high, then lower it. *Repetitions:* Repeat three to five times, then roll to your right side and repeat the entire exercise with your left leg.

31

Exercise No. 15

1 Inhale as you rock your left hip to the side and look around your left arm.

Hip Rock

Aim: To trim your waistline and tone your arms and pectoral muscles.

Starting Position: All fours.

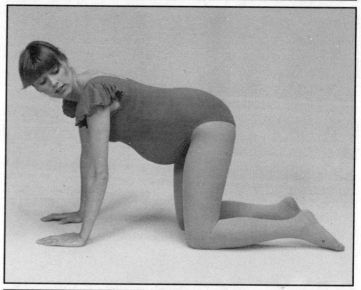

2 Exhale and return to the all-fours position then repeat, rocking your right hip. *Repetitions:* Repeat three times on each side, alternating sides.

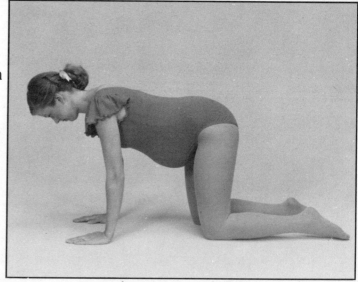

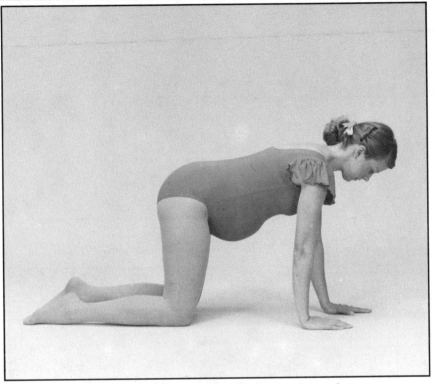

Pelvic Rock
(on all fours)

Aim: To soothe your back muscles, strengthen your arms, lower back and abdominal muscles, and prepare you for delivery.

Starting Position: All fours.

1 Raise your back slightly and hold the position for a few seconds. Return to starting position. *Repetitions:* Repeat three to five times, very slowly.

Note: Be sure to keep your back flat and your elbows, head, and knees still when doing this exercise.

33

Exercise No. 17

Leg Extenders

Aim: To strengthen your lower back, abdominal muscles, pectoral muscles, hamstrings, and buttock muscles.

Starting Position: All fours.

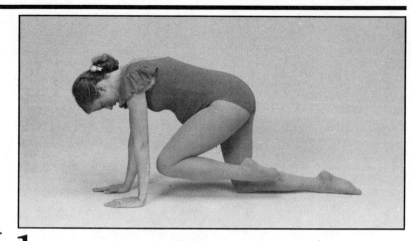

1 Bring your left knee forward, toward your chin.

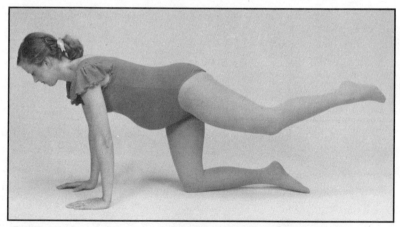

2 Slowly extend your leg back, keeping your knee slightly bent. *Repetitions:* Repeat three times with your left leg, then three times with your right leg. Do a pelvic rock (raise your back slightly), then return to all-fours position.

Note: To avoid any strain as the baby grows, be sure to keep your back flat throughout this exercise.

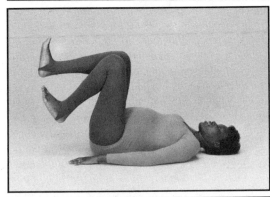

1 Extend your right knee up and straighten your leg toward the ceiling, then return to starting position. Repeat with your left leg.

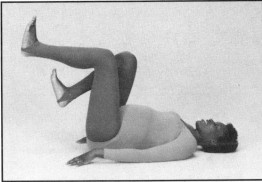

2 Keeping your feet flexed, continue the "flutter" movement ten times with each leg, alternating your legs smoothly.

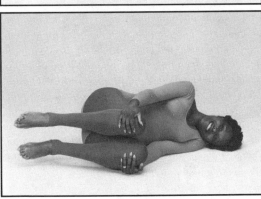

3 Roll to your left side and tighten your vaginal and pelvic muscles as much as you can (the kegel exercise). Hold for a count of five, then relax. Repeat steps 1 and 2, then roll to your right side to kegel. *Repetitions:* Repeat the entire exercise once.

Flex and Flutter

Aim: To strengthen your abdominal muscles, lower back, and legs.

Starting Position: Back tuck, with your feet flexed (toes pointing toward the ceiling).

Exercise No. 19

Open Pelvic Rock

Aim: To strengthen your abdominal muscles, pelvic floor muscles, inner and outer thigh muscles, shoulders, and neck; and to help prepare you for delivery.

Starting Position: Lying on your back, with the soles of your feet together in the butterfly position.

Note: Breathe in, then out as you do the exercise; do not hold your breath. In preparation for delivery, practice relaxing your face during the exercise; but never practice actual pushing.

1 Bring your feet as close to your body as possible, keeping your head up and your shoulder blades off the floor. Press your heels together.

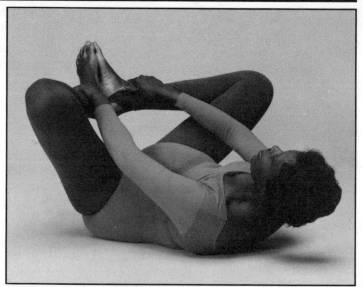

2 Holding your ankles with your hands, pull your ankles toward your chin. At the same time, move your knees outward *only* until you feel a stretch in your inner thigh muscles. *Repetitions:* Repeat three to five times.

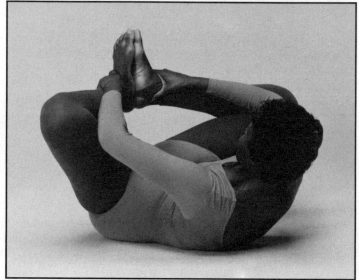

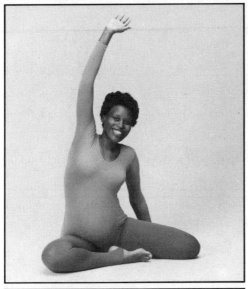

1 Bend to the left and press your right palm slowly toward the ceiling, steadying yourself with your left arm if necessary.

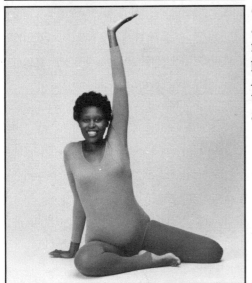

2 Return to starting position, then bend to the right and press your left palm toward the ceiling. *Repetitions:* Repeat five times slowly on each side, alternating sides.

◊ Stretch and Press

Aim: To tone your arms, waist, and lower back.

Starting Position: Side sit or tailor sit.

Note: Breathe in and out normally as you do the exercise.

To do this exercise in water, stand and hold onto the side of the pool.

Exercise No. 21

Leg and Foot Toner

Aim: To stretch and tone your leg and foot muscles and to improve your circulation; done daily, it can help to prevent leg and foot cramps.

Starting Position: Pike sit with your arms behind you and your palms flat on the floor.

To do this exercise in water, stand and hold onto the side of the pool.

1 *Point:* Tighten your leg and buttock muscles. Point your toes, stretch, then relax. *Repetitions:* Repeat five times, then shake out your legs.

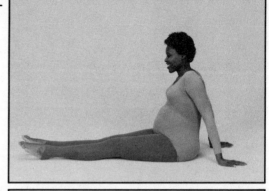

2 *Flex:* Point your toes toward the ceiling. Hold the position as you tighten your leg and buttock muscles, then relax. *Repetitions:* Repeat five times, then shake out your legs.

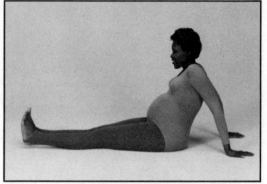

3 *Circle:* Keeping your feet flat on the floor, bend your knees. Lean back and rest on your forearms. Rest your right leg on your left knee and circle your right foot five times to the left, then five times to the right, flexing your foot and pointing your toes as you do so. *Repetitions:* Repeat with your left foot.

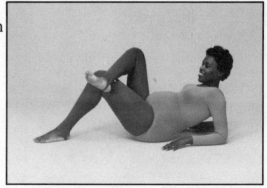

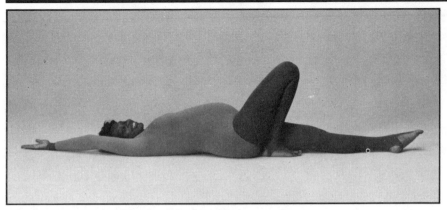

1 Keeping your head and shoulders on the floor, stretch from the fingertips of your right hand to the heel of your left foot; exhale as you do so. Release the stretch, inhale, and return to starting position.

Cross-Body Stretch

Aim: To stretch your entire body.

Starting Position: Lying on your back with your right knee bent and your right foot on the floor, your heel by your hip, your left leg extended, your right arm extended over your head, and your left arm at your side.

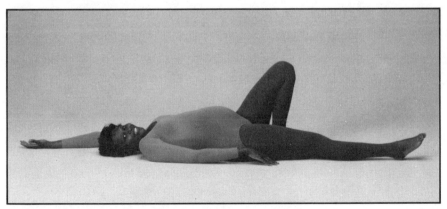

2 Repeat with your left knee bent, your right leg extended, and your left arm extended over your head. *Repetitions:* Repeat the entire exercise three times.

Exercise No. 23

Seat Squeeze

Aim: To strengthen your abdominal and buttock muscles, to increase the flexibility of your back, and to prepare you for delivery.

Starting Position: Hook-lying.

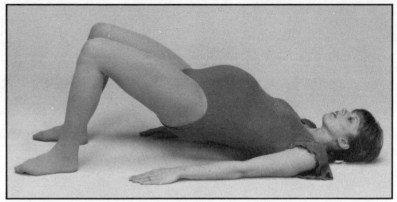

1 "Tuck" your pelvis and pull your abdominal muscles in while raising your hips slightly off the floor, resting your weight on your shoulders. (To avoid putting pressure on your neck, do not raise your hips too high.) Tighten your buttock muscles as much as you can, then release.

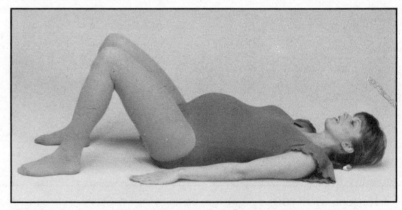

2 Slowly lower your hips to the floor to starting position. *Repetitions:* Repeat five times, then *roll to your side and come to a stand.*

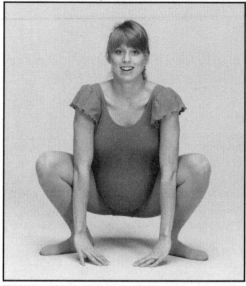

1 Squat, placing your hands on the floor between your legs.

Squats

Aim: To strengthen your inner and outer thigh muscles and to prepare you for pushing during delivery.

Starting Position: Standing with your legs apart and your hands on your hips, with feet pointed out and your knees bent so that your hips are at knee level.

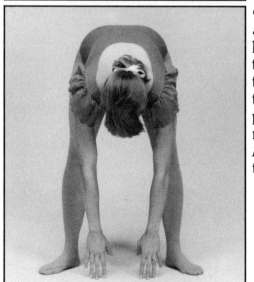

2 Straighten your legs as much as you can, keeping your feet flat on the floor and your hands touching or reaching toward the floor. Hold this position, then relax and return to starting position. *Repetitions:* Repeat five times.

Note: Never practice actual pushing when doing this exercise.

Exercise No. 25

Breathe ◊ and Lunge

Aim: To strengthen your hips and leg muscles.

Starting Position: Standing with your hands on your hips and your feet two to three feet apart.

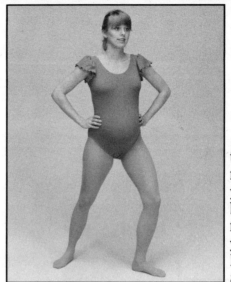

1 Take a deep breath and slowly step forward and to the left with your left foot. Exhale as you bend your left knee, shifting your body weight onto your left foot while striving to keep your right leg extended. Lunge as deeply as comfort allows.

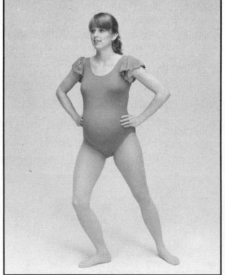

2 Pause, inhale, and return to the center with both feet facing forward. Pivot your right foot out, bend your right knee, shift your weight, and lunge to your right side. *Repetitions:* Repeat five to ten times on each side.

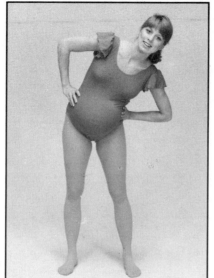

1 Moving from your waist, bend to the left.

⬥Trunk Benders

Aim: To increase the flexibility of your waist, trunk, and lower back.

Starting Position: Standing with your back straight and your hands on your hips.

Note: Never bend backward.

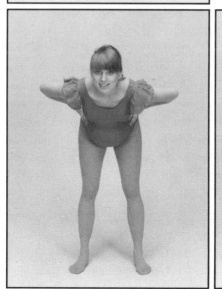

2 Bend forward.

3 Bend to the right, then return to starting position. *Repetitions:* Repeat five times to the left, then five times to the right.

Exercise No. 27

Arm Series 💧

Aim: To strengthen your upper and lower arms, wrists, and pectoral muscles.

Starting Position: Standing with your feet shoulders'-width apart and your arms in cross position.

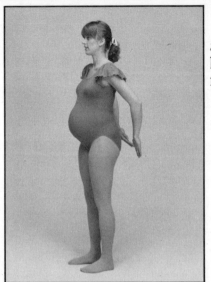

1 *Push Backs:* Turn your palms toward your back and gently press up and back. *Repetitions:* Repeat five times.

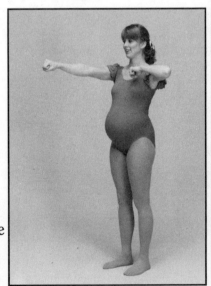

1 *Arm Punches:* Make fists. Punch forward five times, alternating arms. Punch over your head five times, alternating arms.

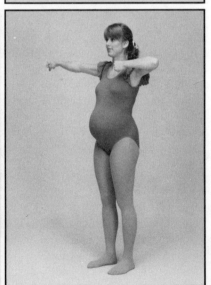

2 Punch out to your sides five times, alternating arms.

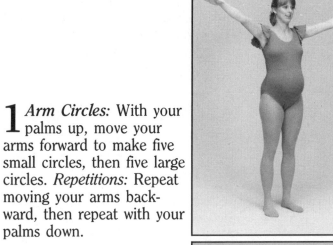

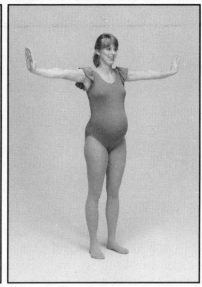

1 *Arm Circles:* With your palms up, move your arms forward to make five small circles, then five large circles. *Repetitions:* Repeat moving your arms backward, then repeat with your palms down.

1 *Wrist Flexors:* Moving only your wrists, point your fingertips toward the ceiling, then toward the floor. *Repetitions:* Repeat five times.

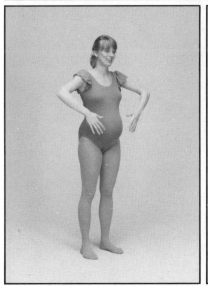

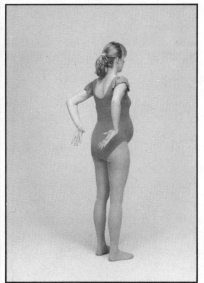

1 *Scarecrow:* With your palms facing backward, spread your fingers. Keeping your upper arms at shoulder height, bend your arms at the elbows and swing your arms in front of your body, then return to starting position. *Repetitions:* Repeat five times.

1 *Back Sweeper:* With your palms facing backward, bend your arms at the elbows and try to bring your fingertips together behind your back, then return to starting position. *Repetitions:* Repeat five times slowly.

Exercise No. 27

Arm Series ⟡

Aim: To strengthen your upper and lower arms, wrists, and pectoral muscles.

Starting Position: Standing with your feet shoulders'-width apart and your arms in cross position.

1 *Elbow Flex:* With your palms up, make fists. Bring your fists to your shoulders, then continue to move them downward and outward in an arc.

2 With your hands still fisted, turn your wrists toward the ceiling.

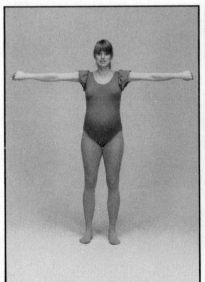

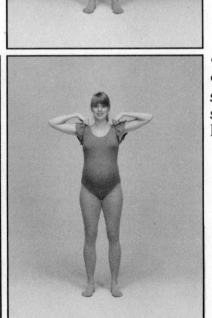

3 Bend your elbows and touch your fists to your shoulders, then return to starting position. *Repetitions:* Repeat five times.

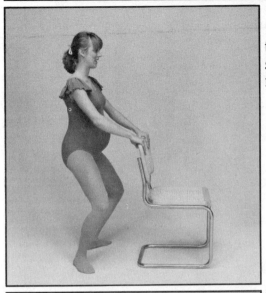

1 Slowly bend both knees, pressing your feet into the floor as if to sit on a stool. Hold the position for five seconds.

◊ Standing Thigh Stretch

Aim: To tone your entire body, especially your legs and inner thighs.

Starting Position: Standing with your legs apart and your toes pointing out.

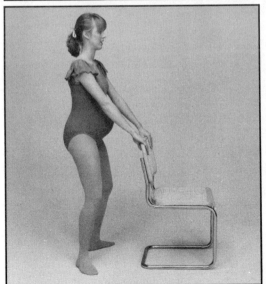

2 Slowly stretch up, keeping your legs tight and your feet flat on the floor as you return to starting position. *Repetitions:* Repeat five times.

Note: Balance against a chair, wall, or bar for support if balance is a problem.

Exercise No. 29

Wall 🌢 Push-Ups

Aim: To strengthen your shoulders and pectoral muscles, and to develop the arm muscles that you use in pushing during delivery.

Starting Position: Standing an arm's length or further from a wall, with your legs comfortably apart.

1 Place your hands on the wall, with your fingertips pointed in and your elbows parallel to the floor.

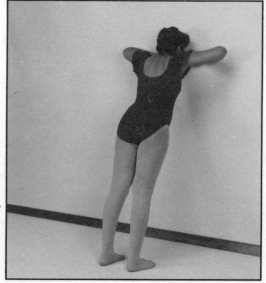

2 Keeping your feet flat on the floor, slowly move toward the wall, inhaling as you do so. Exhale as you slowly push up from the wall. *Repetitions:* Do ten or twenty push-ups.

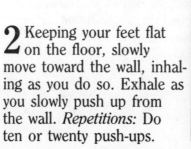

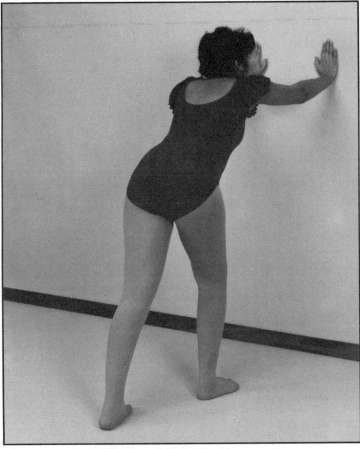

⬦Calf Stretch

Aim: To stretch your calves in preparation for the walking portion of the exercise routine.

Starting Position: Standing with your hands on the wall, your toes pointed forward, and your hips pressed forward.

1 Put your right foot forward with your knee bent, and stretch your left leg behind you (keep both heels on the floor). Keeping your lower back flat, hold a comfortable stretch for fifteen seconds. Do not bounce. Return to starting position. *Repetitions:* Repeat with your left foot forward.

Exercise No. 31

Skier's Sit ◊

Aim: To strengthen your legs, abdominal muscles, and lower back.

Starting Position: Standing with your back against a wall.

1 Bend your knees and slide your upper body down. "Sit" with your thighs at a right angle to the wall, as if you were sitting on a stool. Press the small of your back firmly against the wall. (This is a great time to practice kegels.) Hold this position for twenty to forty-five seconds.

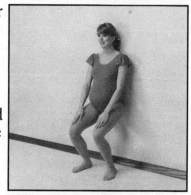

2 Lean forward and place your hands on your knees, then slowly straighten your back. Straighten your knees slowly and return to a standing position.

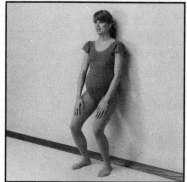

Walking ◊

Aim: To strengthen your cardiovascular system and your legs.

1 Walk briskly. Strive for fifteen to twenty minutes of walking with your heart rate at between fifty and seventy percent of your maximum target heart rate. (See pages 8 to 10 for information about the cardio-vascular system and target heart rate.)

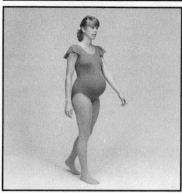

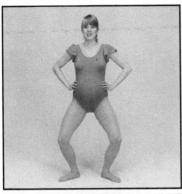

1 *Side-to-side sway:* Sway from side to side, keeping your hips and shoulders in vertical alignment. *Repetitions:* Repeat five times.

⬦ Plié Series

Aim: To tone your legs, waist, buttock muscles, and lower back.

Starting Position: Standing with your feet shoulders'- width apart, with your pelvis tucked, your abdominal muscles pulled in, your knees flexed, and your toes and knees aligned.

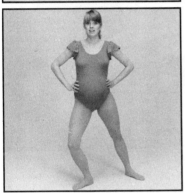

2 *Stride sway:* Keeping your feet shoulders'-width apart, take one step forward with your left foot. Sway forward and back, keeping your heels on the floor. *Repetitions:* Repeat ten times, then repeat ten times with your right foot.

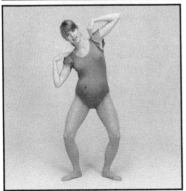

3 *Elbow-hip sway:* Place your hands on your shoulders and lower your right elbow to your right hip, then return to upright position. Lower your left elbow to your left hip, then return to starting position. *Repetitions:* Repeat ten times, alternating sides.

To do this exercise in water, stand in shallow water.

Exercise No. 33

Backache Relievers

Aim: To stretch your lower back, inner thighs, and pectoral muscles.

Starting Position: Tailor sit.

1 Lean forward from the hips until you feel a comfortable stretch while hugging yourself. Do not initiate the forward move from the head; you could strain your lower back.

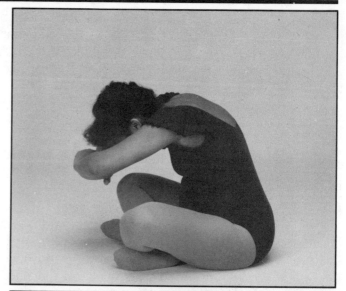

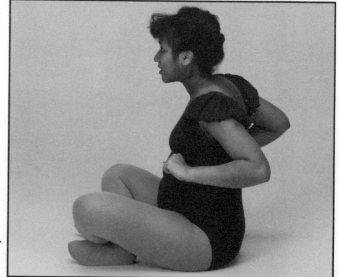

2 Draw your elbows back. *Repetitions:* Repeat three to five times.

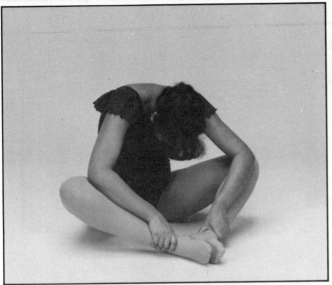

1 Inhale, then exhale as you pull in your abdomen, lower your head as close to your feet as you can, and press your knees toward the floor.

Sitting
Pelvic Stretch

Aim: To strengthen your pelvic floor and inner thighs.

Starting Position: Butterfly sit, holding your ankles.

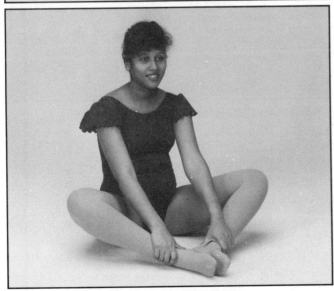

2 Return to starting position. *Repetitions:* Repeat five times.

Exercise No. 35

Thigh Roll

Aim: To tone your waistline, hips, outer thighs, and buttock muscles.

Starting Position: Pike sit.

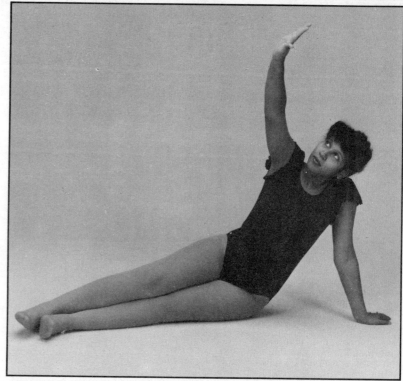

1 Place your left hand to your side to support your weight. Keeping your left hip on the floor, roll to the left, slightly raising your right hip off the floor as you do so. Press your left palm toward the ceiling as you bend to the left. *Repetitions:* Repeat three to five times on each side, alternating sides, rolling slowly.

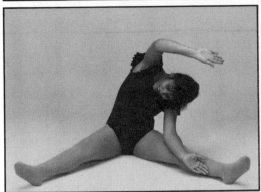

1 Bring your left arm forward to the inside of your left leg so that your elbow is beside your knee and your fingertips are beside your heel. At the same time, bring your right arm over your head and bend to the left.

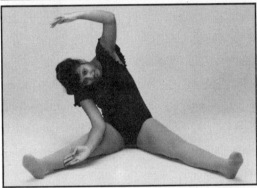

2 Bend forward at the center of your body, holding your chest as close to the floor as possible, then bend to the right.

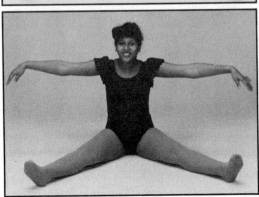

3 Return to starting position and do a swan breath (inhale through your nose while moving your arms upward, then exhale through your mouth while bringing your arms down). *Repetitions:* Repeat the entire exercise five times.

Lateral Straddle Stretch

Aim: To tone your shoulders, arms, hips, quadriceps, calves, buttocks, and waist.

Starting Position: Straddle sit, with your toes pointed comfortably and your arms in cross position.

Exercise No. 37

Hamstring Straddle Stretch

Aim: To stretch your hamstrings and tone your legs, buttocks, arms, and shoulders.

Starting Position: Straddle sit, with your toes pointed comfortably and your arms at your sides.

1 Lean left from your hip and stretch as far forward as you can, looking over your left foot.

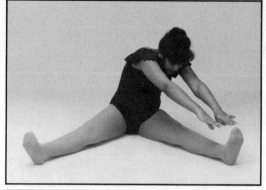

2 Bend forward at the center of your body, holding your chest as close to the floor as possible.

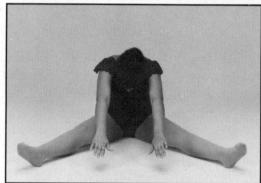

3 Bend to the right, then return to starting position and do a swan breath (inhale through your nose while moving your arms upward, then exhale through your mouth while bringing your arms down). *Repetitions:* Repeat the entire exercise five times.

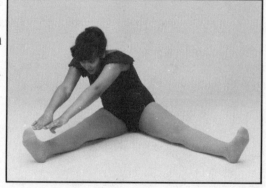

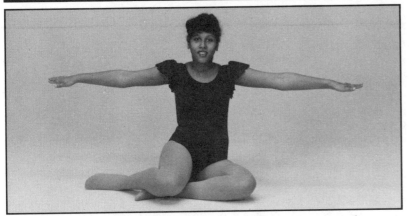

1 Begin with your arms in cross position. Turn to the left, placing your left arm on your left knee as you do so. Placing your left arm behind you for support, look over your left shoulder.

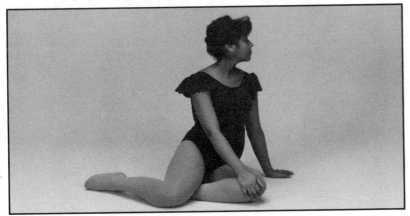

2 Hold the position for five seconds, then return to starting position (with your arms in cross position). *Repetitions:* Repeat three times slowly. Then side-sit with your legs to the left and repeat three times, looking over your right shoulder.

Shoulder Turns

Aim: To increase flexibility in your waist and back, soothe your ribs, and tone your arms and shoulders.

Starting Position: Side sit or a comfortable variation, with your legs to your right side.

Exercise No. 39

Baby-Go-Round

Aim: To relax your neck, shoulders, and back, and to soothe your ribs.

Starting Position: Tailor sit.

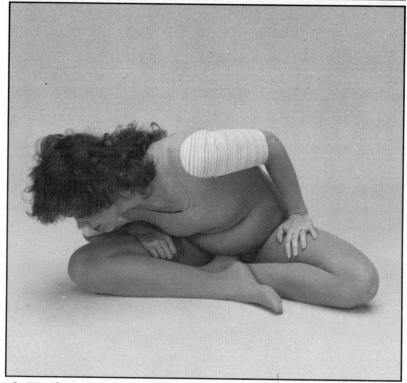

1 Bend your body, head, and shoulders to the right, forward, and to the left in one continuous circular motion. Reverse the circle to the left. *Repetitions:* Alternating directions, do two circles in each direction.

Note: Circle slowly, and never bend backward.

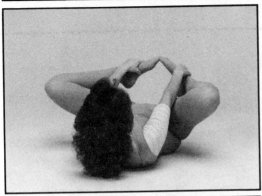

1 Open your knees wide, place your toes together, and slide your hands down to your ankles.

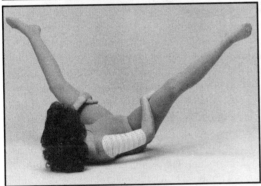

2 Pull your feet close to your body, then slowly straighten your legs out to a V position. Hold the position for a few seconds. Do not bounce.

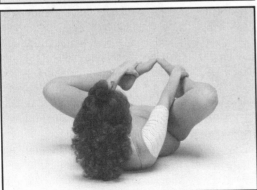

3 Keeping your knees open wide, bring your toes back together, then return to starting position. *Repetitions:* Repeat five times.

V-Stretch

Aim: To tone and strengthen your abdominal muscles, legs, feet, and especially your inner thighs.

Starting Position: Back tuck.

Exercise No. 41

Lower Back Roll

Aim: To massage your lower back and stretch your inner thighs.

Starting Position: Back tuck.

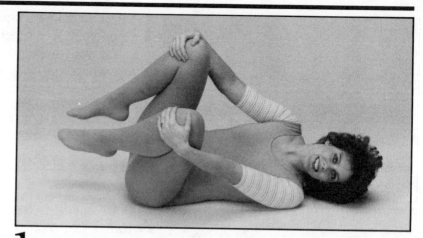

1 Slowly roll to the left.

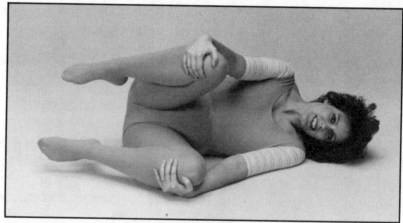

2 Open your legs far enough to feel a stretch in your inner thighs and to create the need to roll to the right, then do so. *Repetitions:* Roll from side to side three to five times (the rolling motion will massage your lower back).

Note: If this exercise hurts your tailbone or bothers you in any way, do it more slowly or stop. You can try it again after your baby is born.

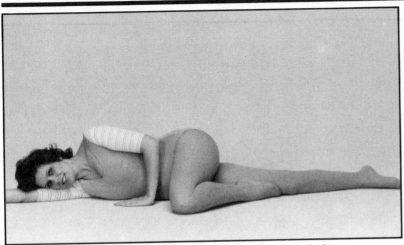

1 Bring your left knee over your right side, shifting your weight to your left hip as you do so.

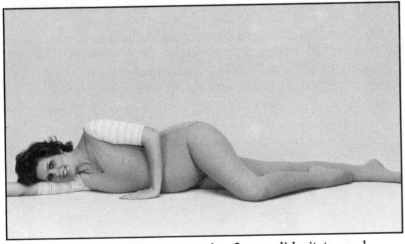

2 Keeping your left knee on the floor, glide it toward your chest and back down until your leg is almost straight. *Repetitions:* Repeat three times on each side.

Knee Gliders

Aim: To relax your lower back, hips, and buttock muscles.

Starting Position: Lying on your right side with your head resting comfortably on your arm, and with your hips and knees slightly bent.

Exercise No. 43

Body Relaxation

Aim: To relax you.

Starting Position: Lying on your left side.

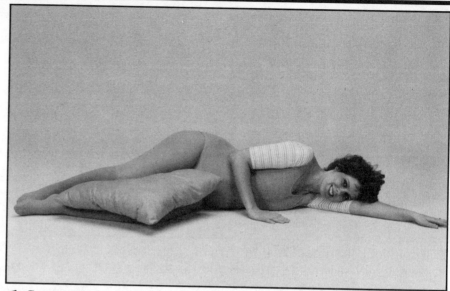

1 Concentrate on something or somewhere very peaceful. Close your eyes and take deep breaths. In the following order, relax your *feet, legs, back, arms, neck, and face.* After you feel totally relaxed and peaceful, open your eyes, roll to all fours, and slowly stand up.

Note: Be sure to keep your face calm during this exercise. During delivery, many women distort their faces; doing this not only misplaces energy, but can result in broken capillaries in the face.

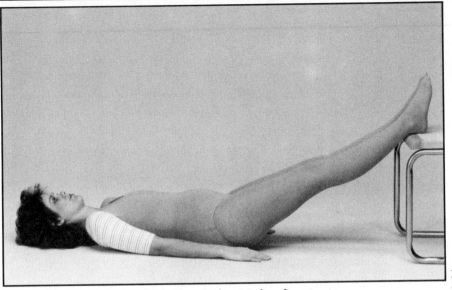

Leg Elevations

Aim: To prevent swelling and improve the circulation in your legs.

Starting Position: Lying flat on your back with your feet flat against a wall or resting on a chair.

1 Lie flat with your feet up, and rest for five to ten minutes. Roll to your side, sit for a moment to prevent light-headedness, then stand up. Try to elevate your legs for at least one-half hour per day, preferably for five or ten minutes in several sessions.

Note: Your legs need to be elevated only above your heart.

Chapter Two
Focus on Delivery

This chapter focuses on the period just before and just after the birth of your baby. It includes exercises to help you prepare for the possibility of a cesarean delivery and two sets of exercises to do in the hospital—one if you have given birth vaginally and the other if you have had a cesarean.

The best time to start your postpartum exercises is immediately after delivery or as soon as you feel up to it, provided your doctor has given his or her permission. You can begin getting back into shape while you are still in the hospital. Regardless of what kind of delivery you have, exercising within the first week after delivery helps relieve discomfort. To avoid any strain on your spine or any additional stretching of muscles, do the exercises in this chapter in your bed and use pillows to make yourself as comfortable as possible.

Human Relations

Labor is hard work. You can begin to prepare for getting the help you need during labor and delivery by encouraging your husband to read books about pregnancy and to participate with you in whatever prenatal classes or groups you are involved in. You need not be committed to any specific approach to delivery to benefit from the information and support that prenatal classes provide.

You and your husband also will probably want to learn about the possible complications of delivery that may require medical intervention (such as cesarean delivery) and special medications. Knowing about and discussing these issues together before delivery can help reduce the fear and mystery associated with them.

Another topic to focus on is breathing techniques. These techniques are not only crucial during delivery, but are also an important component of many prenatal exercises. A number of breathing exercises and techniques are covered in prenatal classes, as well as in many books about pregnancy and labor (see pages 15 to 17 in this book for breathing exercises).

After the delivery, you may be tempted to pay all of your attention to your newborn. As important as the new baby is, you and your partner deserve attention from one another as well.

Cesarean Delivery

Any unforeseen procedure such as an emergency cesarean can totally alter the experience of giving birth, but it need not destroy the beauty of the moment. When complications arise, the ability of a doctor to immediately reach your baby, if it becomes necessary, is a miraculous option for a healthy delivery.

A large percentage of cesarean deliveries are performed as emergencies. Many women find themselves unprepared because they haven't anticipated the possibility that a cesarean might be necessary to ensure a safe delivery in their particular situation. It is far better to be aware of the possibility of a surgical delivery than to be alarmed by the sudden necessity for one. Contact your hospital or doctor for information about cesarean delivery and classes in which cesarean birth is discussed.

Whether you know you will have a cesarean delivery or not, it is best to prepare for the possibility. The cesarean preparation exercise routine that follows is intended to help you to do so.

Exercise No. 1

Simple Breaths

Aim: To teach you to breathe down into your diaphragm.

Starting Position: Tailor sit, with your hands on your stomach and the fingertips of your middle fingers touching lightly.

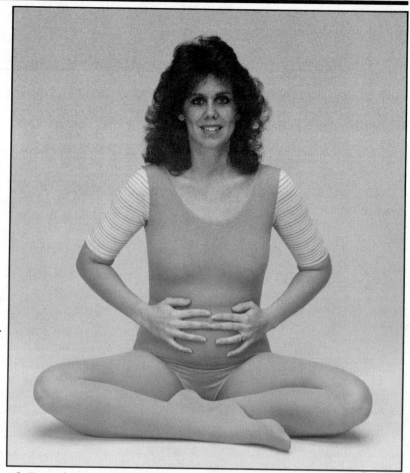

1 Breathing in through your nose, bring air into your lungs and allow it to push your stomach outward. Your fingertips should move apart slightly as your stomach expands. Hold your breath for a count of five, then slowly exhale (this will bring your fingertips back together). *Repetitions:* Repeat slowly three to five times.

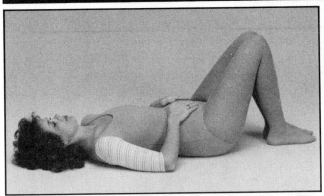

1 Press the sides of your hands firmly into your lower abdomen to practice supporting a vertical incision.

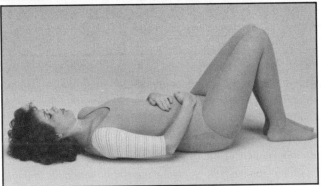

2 Press the sides of your hands firmly into your lower abdomen to practice supporting a horizontal incision.

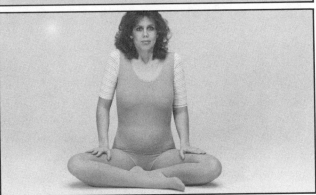

3 *Huffing:* Breathe in deeply and sharply, then force air out and say "haa." *Coughing:* Cough hard (if this is too difficult, continue to practice huffing).

Huffing/ Coughing

Aim: To strengthen your diaphragm and make it easier to cough after surgery (particularly after receiving a general anesthetic).

Starting Position: Hook-lying.

Exercise No. 3

Tuck and Pull

Aim: To strengthen your abdominal muscles and lengthen your lumbar muscles; also helps reduce backache.

Starting Position: Hook-lying or standing.

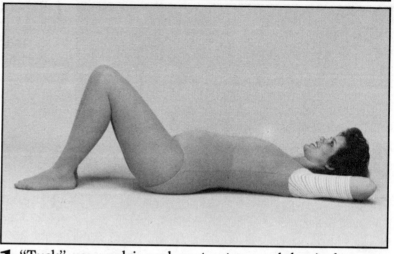

1 "Tuck" your pelvis and contract your abdominal muscles.

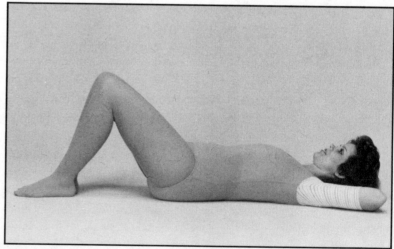

2 Hold the position for several seconds, then release. *Repetitions:* Repeat eight to ten times.

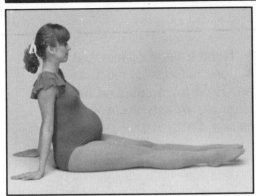

1 *Point:* Tighten your leg and buttock muscles, then point your toes, stretch, and pause. Relax. *Repetitions:* Repeat five times, then shake out your legs.

Leg and Foot Toner

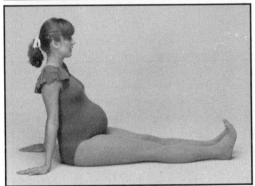

2 *Flex:* Point your toes toward the ceiling. Hold the position as you tighten your leg and buttock muscles, then relax. *Repetitions:* Repeat five times, then shake out your legs.

Aim: To tone your leg and foot muscles and to improve your circulation; done daily, it can help prevent leg and foot cramps.

Starting Position: Pike sit with your palms flat on the floor behind you.

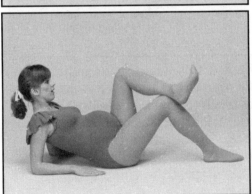

3 *Circle:* Keeping your feet flat on the floor, bend your knees, then lean back and rest on your forearms. Rest your left leg on your right knee and circle your left foot five times to the left, then five times to the right, flexing your foot and pointing your toes as you do so. *Repetitions:* Repeat with your right leg.

Kegels

Flex and Flutter

Aim: To strengthen your abdominal muscles, lower back, and legs.

Starting Position: Back tuck, with your feet flexed (toes pointing toward the ceiling).

Aim: To strengthen your pelvic floor muscles.

Starting Position: Standing, sitting, or lying down.

Note: Intermix kegels with other exercises during your exercise routine.

1 Tighten your vaginal and pelvic floor muscles as much as you can. Hold for a count of five, then relax. *Repetitions:* Repeat several times a day.

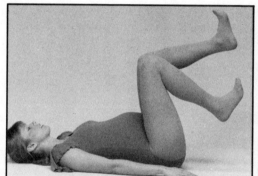

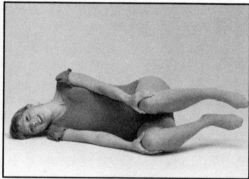

1 Extend your right knee up and straighten your leg toward the ceiling, then return to starting position. Repeat with your left leg. Keeping your feet flexed, continue the "flutter" movement ten times with each leg, alternating your legs smoothly.

2 Roll to your left side and tighten your vaginal and pelvic muscles as much as you can (the kegel exercise). Hold for a count of five, then relax. Repeat steps 1 and 2, rolling to your right side to kegel. *Repetitions:* Repeat the entire exercise once.

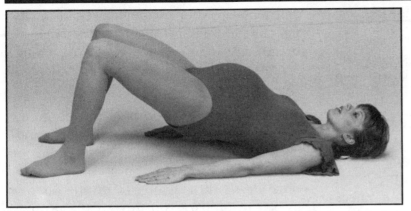

1 "Tuck" your pelvis and pull your abdominal muscles in while raising your hips slightly off the floor, resting your weight on your shoulders. (To avoid putting pressure on your neck, do not raise your hips too high.) Tighten your buttock muscles as much as you can, then release.

Seat Squeeze

Aim: To strengthen your abdominal and buttock muscles, increase the flexibility of your back, and to prepare you for delivery.

Starting Position: Hook-lying.

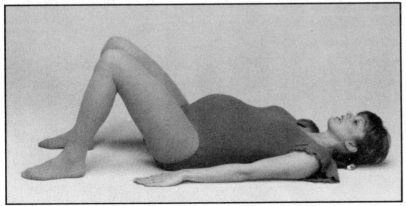

2 Slowly lower your hips to the floor to the starting position. *Repetitions:* Repeat five times, then roll to your side and come to a stand.

71

Hospital Exercise Routine Following a Cesarean Delivery

Tightening your abdominal muscles slowly as soon after surgery as possible will help speed up your recovery.

After the delivery, take a couple of deep breaths, bend your feet, wiggle your toes, and tighten and relax your leg muscles. On your second or third day in the hospital, lie on your side with both your knees bent. This will encourage the natural progress of gas through your intestines. To help eliminate gas, lie on your side and massage your abdominal region to expel gas naturally. You can also try the breathing exercise described below under "Hints for Recovery from a Cesarean Delivery."

A day or two after you have started doing the deep breathing and muscle tightening exercises, add the postpartum exercises on pages 73 to 76. After you go home, continue doing these exercises on the floor or in bed to prepare you to start the postpartum exercise routine (pages 87 to 126).

Hints for Recovering from a Cesarean Delivery

• Do no heavy lifting for a minimum of three weeks following delivery. Limit lifting to ten to fifteen percent of your body weight.

• Before coughing, sneezing, or laughing, support the incision with your hands (see page 67).

• Nursing will speed your recovery, but your milk may be delayed for a couple of days. Find a comfortable position and have patience; it will come.

• Return to a regular fitness routine as soon after delivery as your doctor will allow.

• To help eliminate gas, lie on your side and massage your abdominal region to expel gas naturally. Try this exercise for gas pains:

1. Take a big breath in, then blow it out.
2. Take another big breath in and blow it out.
3. Take a big breath in, then blow it out slowly while tightening and contracting your abdominal muscles.
4. Take a big breath in and blow it out. Take two or three breaths at a time periodically, as soon as the first twinge of a gas pain appears.

Postpartum Breathing

Aim: To help you breathe down into your diaphragm.

Starting Position: Hook-lying in bed, with your legs slightly apart and your hands on your stomach with your fingertips touching.

1 Breathe in through your nose, bringing air into your diaphragm. Hold your breath to a count of five, then slowly exhale to a count of five. *Repetitions:* Repeat three or four times.

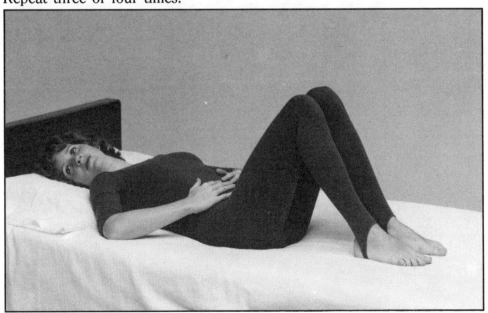

Exercise No. 2

1 *Point:* Point your toes and tighten your abdominal, leg, and buttock muscles. Relax. *Repetitions:* Repeat ten times.

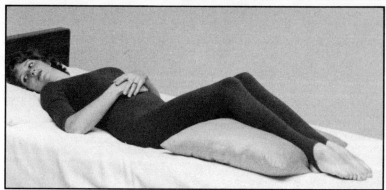

Leg and Foot Toner

Aim: To stretch and tone your legs and foot muscles and to improve your circulation; done daily, it can help prevent leg and foot cramps.

Starting Position: Lying flat on your back in bed, with a pillow under your knees and your legs out straight in front of you.

2 *Flex:* In the same position, point your toes toward the ceiling. Hold the position, then relax. *Repetitions:* Repeat ten times. Shake out your legs.

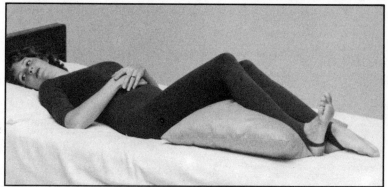

3 *Circle:* In the same position, circle your right foot five times to the right, then five times to the left. *Repetitions:* Repeat with your left foot.

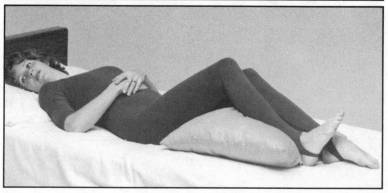

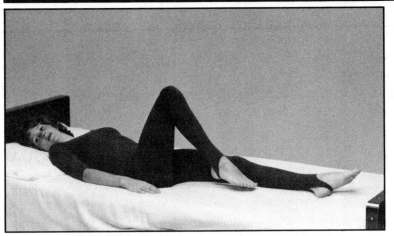

1 Bend your right knee slowly, then straighten it. Bend and straighten your left knee. *Repetitions:* Repeat five to ten times on each leg, alternating legs.

Knee Bends

Aim: To tone your legs.

Starting Position: Lying flat on your back in bed.

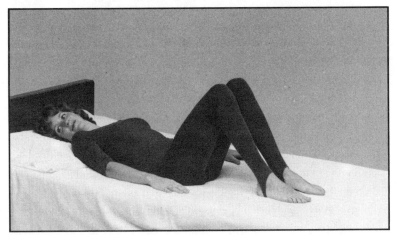

1 Tighten your vaginal and pelvic floor muscles as much as you can. Hold for a count of five, then relax. *Repetitions:* Repeat several times a day.

Kegels

Aim: To strengthen your pelvic floor muscles.

Starting Position: Lying in bed (or in the bathtub) in a comfortable position.

Exercise Nos. 5 and 6

Pelvic Rock

Aim: To soothe your lower back and strengthen your abdominal muscles.

Starting Position: Hook-lying in bed, with your legs slightly apart and your arms in cross position.

Seat Squeeze

Aim: To strengthen your abdominal and buttock muscles and increase the flexibility of your back.

Starting Position: Hook-lying in bed.

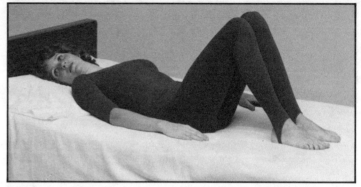

1 Relax your back and press your lower back into the bed as you "tuck" your pelvis and contract your abdominal muscles. Relax. *Repetitions:* Repeat five times slowly.

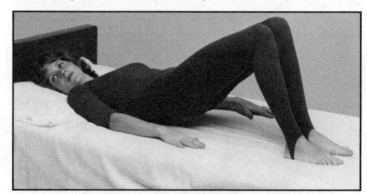

1 "Tuck" your pelvis and contract your abdominal muscles while raising your hips off the bed, resting your weight on your shoulders. Tighten your buttock muscles as much as you can. Hold the position, then relax and slowly lower your hips to starting position. *Repetitions:* Repeat once.

Hospital Exercise Routine Following a Vaginal Delivery

Most women experience labor-like contractions, called afterbirth pains, twenty-four to forty-eight hours after the birth of second or subsequent babies. If you are breastfeeding, the pains may be stronger. They can occur at any time, but especially each time you breastfeed your baby. Try the following breathing exercise when you are lying in bed to help relieve afterbirth pains and gas pains:

1. Take a big breath and blow it out.

2. Take another big breath and blow it out.

3. Take a third breath in and as you blow it out, contract your abdominal muscles.

4. Take a big breath and blow it out. Repeat the exercise two or three times, whenever you feel afterbirth pains or gas pains.

As soon as possible after delivery, start the hospital exercise routine on pages 78 to 83.

Lying On Your Stomach

Aim: To help your uterus return to normal.

Starting Position: Roll over onto your stomach.

Note: For comfort, you may want to put a pillow under your chest and head, and rest on your folded arms.

Kegels

Aim: To strengthen your pelvic floor muscles.

Starting Position: Lying in bed (or in the bathtub) in a comfortable position.

Note: If you kegel each time you sit down, it will help you immensely in the weeks after delivery.

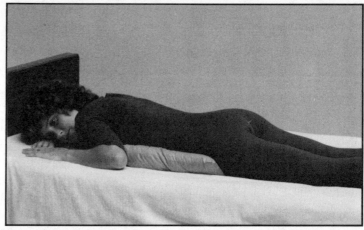

1 Try to spend at least a half-hour per day on your stomach reading, sleeping, or relaxing.

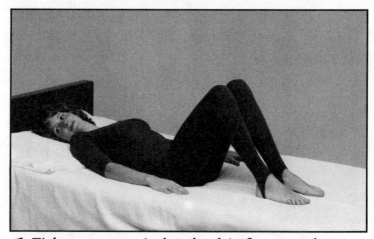

1 Tighten your vaginal and pelvic floor muscles as much as you can. Hold for a count of five, then relax. *Repetitions:* Repeat several times a day.

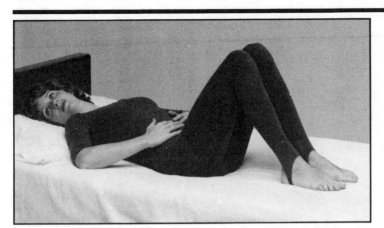

1 Breathe in through your nose, bringing air into your diaphragm. Hold your breath to a count of five, then slowly exhale to a count of five. *Repetitions:* Repeat three to five times.

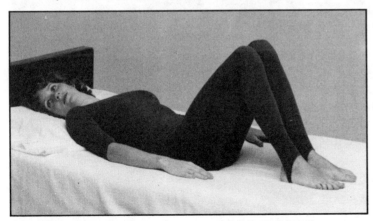

1 Relax your back and press your lower back into the bed as you "tuck" your pelvis and contract your abdominal muscles. Relax. *Repetitions:* Repeat five times slowly.

Note: The next day, continue to do the two exercises on the previous page, and add the following four exercises.

Postpartum Breathing

Aim: To help you breathe down into your diaphragm.

Starting Position: Hook-lying in bed, with your legs slightly apart and your hands on your stomach with your fingertips touching.

Pelvic Rock

Aim: To soothe your lower back and strengthen your abdominal muscles.

Starting Position: Hook-lying in bed, with your legs slightly apart and your arms in cross position.

Exercise No. 5

Knee Bends

Aim: To tone your legs.

Starting Position: Lying flat on your back in bed.

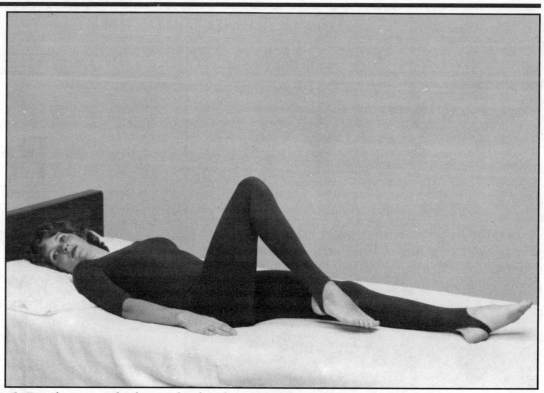

1 Bend your right knee slowly, then straighten it. Bend and straighten your left knee. *Repetitions:* Repeat five to ten times on each leg, alternating legs.

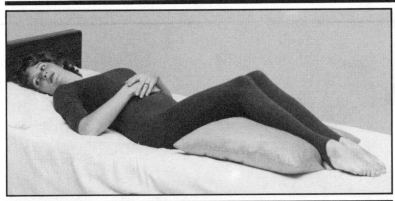

1 *Point:* Point your toes and tighten your abdominal, leg, and buttock muscles. Relax. *Repetitions:* Repeat ten times.

Exercise No. 6

Leg and Foot Toner

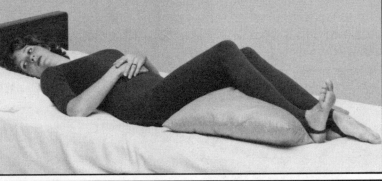

2 *Flex:* In the same position, point your toes toward the ceiling. Hold the position, then relax. *Repetitions:* Repeat ten times. Shake out your legs.

Aim: To stretch and tone your leg and foot muscles and to improve your circulation; done daily, it can help prevent leg and foot cramps.

Starting Position: Lying flat on your back in bed, with a pillow under your knees and your legs out straight in front of you.

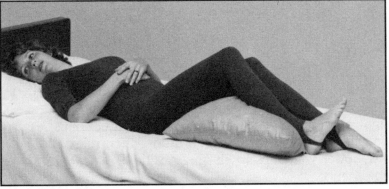

3 *Circle:* In the same position, circle your right foot five times to the right, then five times to the left. *Repetitions:* Repeat with your left foot.

81

Exercise Nos. 7 and 8

On the third day, continue with the exercises on pages 78 to 81 and add the following three exercises. After you're home, continue doing these exercises on the floor to prepare you to start the postpartum exercise routine.

Back Tucks

Aim: To strengthen your lower back and buttock muscles.

Starting Position: Lying flat on your back in bed.

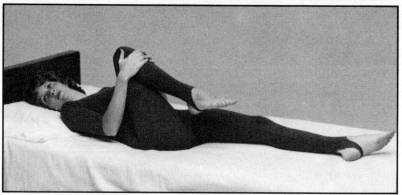

1 Keeping your back flat on the bed, bring one knee up close to your chest and grasp it with your arms, then slowly lower your leg. *Repetitions:* Repeat five times with each leg, alternating legs.

Seat

Squeeze

Aim: To strengthen your abdominal and buttock muscles and increase the flexibility of your back.

Starting Position: Hook-lying on your bed.

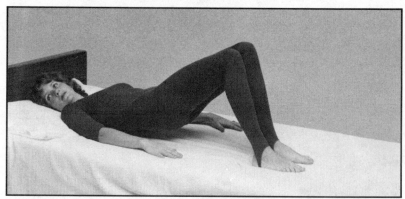

1 "Tuck" your pelvis and pull your abdominal muscles in while raising your hips off the bed, resting your weight on your shoulders. Tighten your buttock muscles as much as you can. Hold the position, then relax and slowly lower your hips to starting position. *Repetitions:* Repeat once.

1 Draw your right leg to your chest.

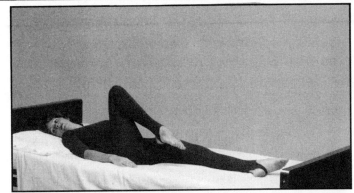

Leg Raisers

2 Extend your leg to the ceiling, pointing your toes as you do so. Press your lower back to the floor.

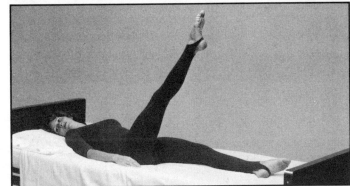

Aim: To strengthen your abdominal and buttock muscles, lower back, and legs.

Starting Position: Hook-lying.

3 Flex your right foot and lower your leg slowly to the floor. *Repetitions:* Repeat three times with each leg, alternating legs.

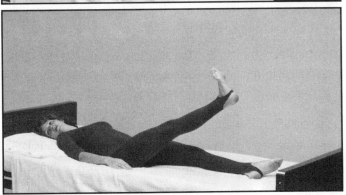

Note: After you are home, continue this exercise routine on the floor at home to prepare you to start the postpartum exercise routine (pages 87 to 126).

Chapter Three
Postpartum Concerns and Exercise Routine

This chapter begins with a discussion of what post-partum adjustment means to both you and your husband and concludes with a postpartum exercise routine that you can begin when you come home from the hospital.

Human Relations

The difficulties of adjusting to a new baby can make the weeks following delivery a very stressful time for the whole family. During the postpartum period, the stress of learning to cope with the demands of a new-born, magnified by being in a state of chronic fatigue, can cause your self-esteem to hit bottom. At the same time, your husband may feel left out, neglected, and jealous of the baby. These feelings, perhaps compounded by fears that he will harm the seemingly delicate baby, can lower his self-esteem as well. When both parents feel this way, the result can be a combination of anger and despair.

This is not to stress the negative aspects of post-baby family life, but rather to emphasize the importance of sharing your concerns with each other during this sometimes trying period. It may help to remember that what all the members of the family need most at this time is caring attention from one other.

Some experts say that the postpartum mother herself needs mothering. Your ability to become attached to and care for your baby may be determined in part by the love and caring you receive from others. Therefore, your husband must be sensitive to this need and make the extra effort to be with you and to support you with his words and deeds.

One study of "postpartum blues" recommends that the new mother take time to relax and separate herself from the events of the day, every day. In order to do this, you will have to ask for help from others, and especially from your husband. It is important that you learn to do so, for by caring for yourself—whether by napping while your husband cares for the baby, soaking in a hot bath, or going shopping for an hour—you will be caring for those close to you, including your baby.

Your husband needs special attention as well. To counteract feelings of being left out, he can take care of the baby for short periods of time when you are not present. By helping out in this way, he can reduce the burden on you while he builds up his competence as a parent. Contact with the baby will also reduce any fears he may have about the delicacy of the newborn, and will help him feel close to both the baby and you. If your husband is feeling neglected from a lack of sexual contact, he may need to discover closeness that is possible without intercourse.

It is also important that you make time to be together as a couple, without your baby. Arranging for competent baby-sitting help will help improve your physical and mental health. Another study of postpartum blues found that among the keys to successful readjustment were continuing to socialize as a couple, though less often than before, and continuing outside interests while limiting outside responsibilities.

The key to getting through the postpartum adjustment period is to share your feelings with your partner and to decide together how to work out problems, instead of holding anger and resentment inside.

A first step might be for you and your husband to talk about what each of you knows and doesn't know about the baby. There is no assurance in our society today that either parent knows anything about caring for a newborn. Your role as parents is just beginning; every few months for the next twenty years, your child will probably present you with a new mystery to solve. The challenge to you and your husband is to learn together and to ask for help.

There is more help available to parents than they usually recognize. Abundant advice can be had not only from books, but also from pediatricians and counselors, teachers and youth workers, and other parents. Sometimes parents lack the self-confidence to ask questions and to seek help; or they may believe that if they join a parenting group, they will be admitting to some fault on their part. Parents need to recognize that it is natural to seek training in the important task of child-rearing. The result will be healthier parents, children, and families.

Postpartum Exercise Routine

After nine months, you probably can't wait to get back into your "normal" clothes. Then, to your disappointment, you find that the dimensions of your hips have changed dramatically, leftover pounds remain to be lost, and your stomach still looks pregnant.

Many women trace lifelong weight problems back to not getting their bodies back into shape after pregnancy. Gynecologists say that doing exercises to strengthen the pelvic floor during and after pregnancy helps prevent possible prolapse of the uterus (i.e., sliding of the uterus down into the vaginal canal) later in

life. It is extremely important to get back into shape as soon after your child's birth as possible by following a program of exercises to strengthen the pelvic floor area. Although your baby's first year of life is a very busy time for you, any delay in taking care of yourself will likely backfire. An out-of-shape, unhappy woman is not as effective a mother as she could be.

As you begin this exercise routine, remember that, first and foremost, you must have patience. You can get back into shape, lose weight, and firm up by exercising—but it won't happen instantly. Also, you may not return to your prepregnancy dimensions or weight, particularly if you are nursing. If you are nursing, add five to ten pounds to your target weight to compensate for retained fluids, etc. This is called your "nursing weight." The time to lose additional weight is after you have finished nursing your baby.

Your postpartum exercise routine will be easier if you have exercised during pregnancy. Be sure to check with your doctor before you start any exercise program. It is extremely important to be sure you have healed and that any bleeding has stopped before doing this postpartum exercise routine.

To chart your progress, you may want to record your weight and measurements when you start, check them six weeks later, and then check them periodically for the next year. Remember—start slowly, then gradually work up to your target heart rate and down to your target weight. And enjoy every little sign of progress!

Note: If you are using this book on your own, rather than in conjunction with a You & Me, Baby exercise class, you'll benefit most from the postpartum exercise routine if you perform it at least three times a week. The exercises are intended to be performed in the order in which they are presented here.

1 Start walking slowly, then lengthen your stride, swinging your arms in an exaggerated motion as you do so. Maintain a rhythm of breathing, and relax.

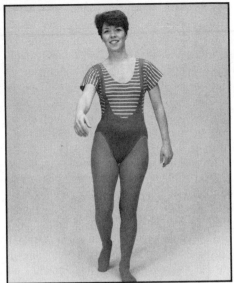

Walking

Aim: To slowly "waken" your body by loosening up your muscles through a series of relaxed leg exercises combined with arm work.

Starting Position: Walking.

2 Alternately raise your right and left knees as you walk, to help loosen your hip flexor muscles.

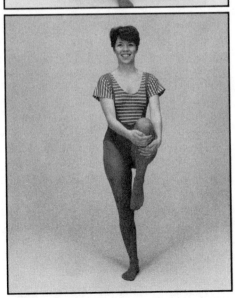

Note: As you walk more briskly, add the arm exercises on the next page.

Exercise No. 2

Walking–
Arm Exercises

Aim: To slowly "waken" your body by loosening up your muscles through a series of relaxed leg exercises combined with arm work.

Starting Position: Walking.

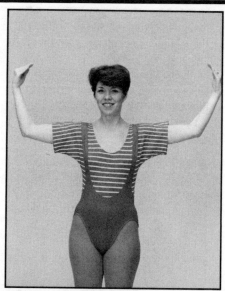

1 Extend your arms at shoulder level.

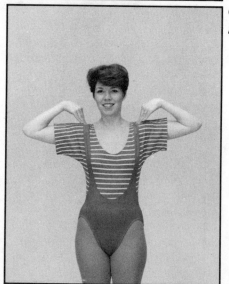

2 Bend your elbows and tap your shoulders.

3 Cross your hands over your head to touch opposite ears.

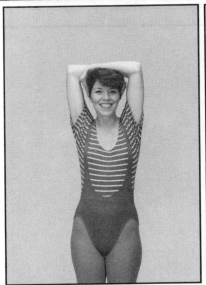

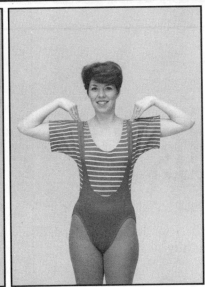

1 *Variation:* Bring your hands to your shoulders.

4 Return your hands to your shoulders and extend your arms again. *Repetitions:* Repeat quickly, to a count of four.

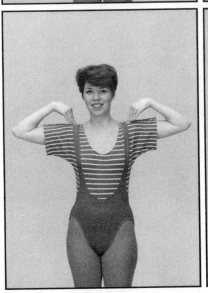

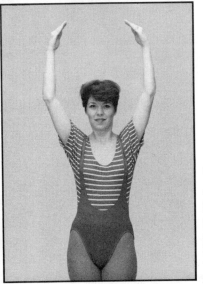

2 Extend your arms upward, return your hands to your shoulders, and extend your arms at shoulder level again. *Repetitions:* Repeat quickly, to a count of four.

Exercise No. 3

Windmills

Aim: To loosen up your arm and shoulder muscles.

Starting Position: Standing with your legs shoulders'-width apart and your knees slightly flexed, with your arms in cross position.

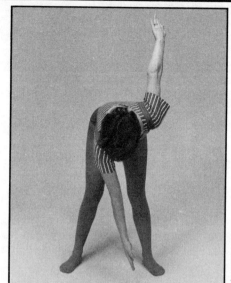

1 Bend at the waist and touch your right hand to your left foot.

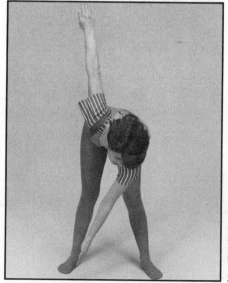

2 Touch your left hand to your right foot. *Repetitions:* Repeat ten to twenty times, alternating sides, then return to starting position.

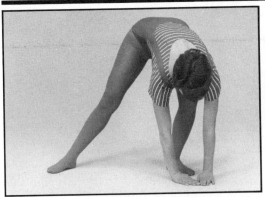

1 Roll your upper body downward gently. Touching your hands to the floor for balance, bend your left knee slowly, straightening your right leg as you shift your weight to your left foot.

Hip Shift and Reach Through

Aim: To loosen up your arm and shoulder muscles.

Starting Position: Standing comfortably with your feet two to three feet apart.

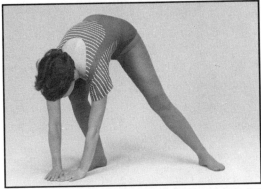

2 Slowly return to the center. Bend your right knee, shifting your weight to your right foot as you extend your left leg.

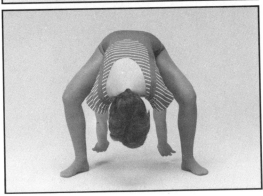

3 Return to center, relax both legs, and reach as far back between your legs as is comfortably possible. *Repetitions:* Repeat the entire exercise two to five times.

Exercise No. 5

Raggedy Ann

Aim: To loosen up and relax your body, particularly your neck, shoulders, and legs. This exercise can be done at any time during the exercise routine.

Starting Position: Standing with your legs slightly apart and your arms above your head.

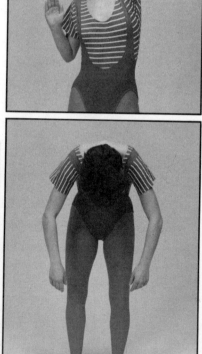

1 Press your left palm toward the ceiling, stretching the entire left side of your body until your left heel rises slightly off the floor. *Repetitions:* Repeat on your right side, then on your left side, then again on your right side.

2 With your knees slightly bent, round your shoulders and raise your arms to shoulder level. Alternately press forward with your left hand, then with your right hand, as if pushing an object away.

3 Keeping your hips aligned with your shoulders, drop your arms forward, drop your chin to your chest, round your shoulders forward, and bend your knees. Hold your body in a slightly flexed position and dangle for five to ten seconds. With your chin on your chest, roll up to starting position. *Repetitions:* Repeat the entire exercise one to three times.

1 *Shoulder Rotations:* Raise your shoulders to your ears. Pull your shoulders back and downward, then up and forward.

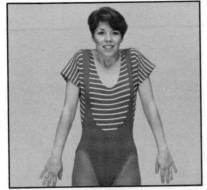

Shoulders

Aim: To loosen up your shoulders and tone your upper arms.

Starting Position: Standing with your feet slightly apart and your arms at your sides; may also be done sitting.

2 With your left shoulder, "draw" three circles forward, then three circles backward. Repeat with your right shoulder. Draw three circles forward with both shoulders, then reverse and draw three circles backward.

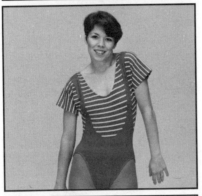

1 *Shoulder Lifts:* Lift your shoulders and roll them forward. With your palms facing out, bring your arms forward until your little fingers touch.

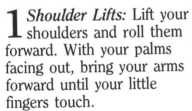

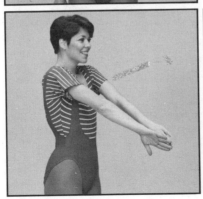

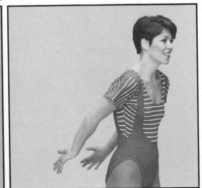

2 Lift your shoulders again and roll them backwards. With your palms still facing out, bring your arms behind your body until you feel the stretch in your shoulders. *Repetitions:* Repeat three times.

Exercise No. 6

Shoulders

Aim: To loosen up your shoulders and tone your upper arms.

Starting Position: Standing with your feet slightly apart and your arms at your sides; may also be done sitting.

Note: Never drop your head and shoulders to the back.

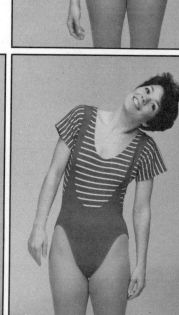

1 *Shoulder Triangles:* Stabilize your abdominal region and tighten your buttocks. Move your head and your right shoulder slightly forward and to the right.

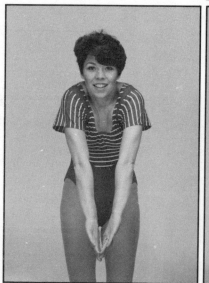

2 Roll both shoulders forward and let your head drop forward slightly.

3 Gently move your head and shoulders forward and to the left, then return to starting position. *Repetitions:* Repeat, moving from left to right.

94

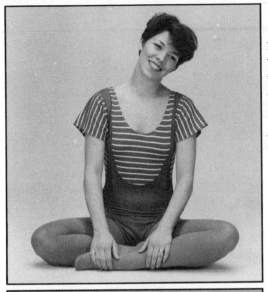

1 Drop your left ear to your left shoulder. Gently roll your head forward to the center of your body, then drop your right ear to your right shoulder and return to starting position. *Repetitions:* Repeat three times in each direction.

Head Arcs

Aim: To loosen up your neck and shoulders.

Starting Position: Tailor sit.

Note: *Do not* roll your head back during the exercise.

Face Exercise

Aim: To tighten your face muscles.

Starting Position: Tailor sit.

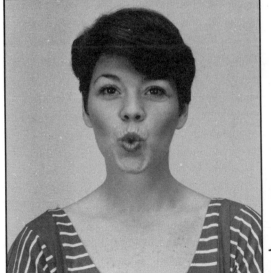

1 Smile, pucker your face, then relax.

Exercise No. 9

Nursing Exercise

Aim: To loosen up your neck and shoulders and stretch your pectoral muscles.

Starting Position: Tailor sit.

1 Clasp your hands behind your back.

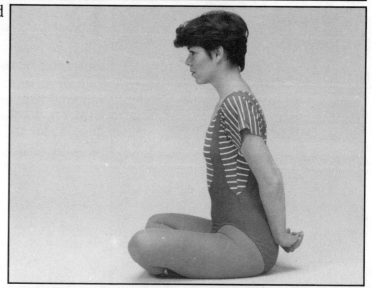

2 Keeping your head centered, lift your arms as you lean forward until you feel a stretch in your pectoral muscles. *Repetitions:* Repeat three to five times.

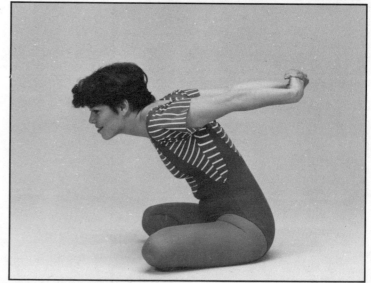

Note: This is an excellent exercise for nursing moms.

1 Holding your right leg, bend your knee toward your chest. Hold onto the outside of your right ankle with one hand and cradle your knee with the other arm, as though you were cradling a baby.

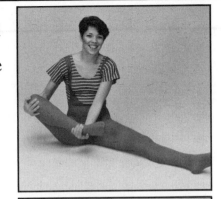

Cradle Stretch

2 Slowly pull your right leg toward your chest. Hold the position for fifteen seconds as you circle your right ankle. *Repetitions:* Repeat with your left leg.

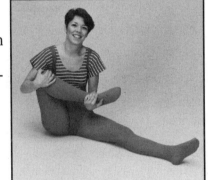

Aim: To tone your neck, shoulders, arms, lower back, hips, legs, and buttocks.

Starting Position: Straddle sit, with your toes pointed.

1 *Variation:* As you cradle your right knee with your right elbow and hold your right calf with your left arm, rock your right leg back and forth and from side to side in a gentle swaying motion.

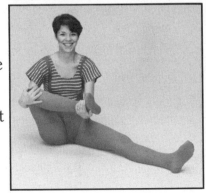

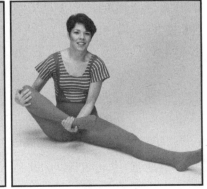

2 Roll your hip socket in a circular motion, three times to the right and three times to the left, striving to keep your left hip bone in the center of rotation. *Repetitions:* Repeat the exercise with your left leg.

Exercise No. 11

Lateral Straddle Stretch

Aim: To tone your shoulders, arms, hips, quadriceps, calves, buttocks, and waist.

Starting Position: Straddle sit, with your toes pointed comfortably and your arms in cross position.

1 Bring your left arm forward to the inside of your left leg so that your elbow is beside your knee and your fingertips are beside your heel. At the same time, bring your right arm over your head and bend to the left.

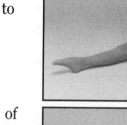

2 Bend forward at the center of your body, holding your chest as close to the floor as possible.

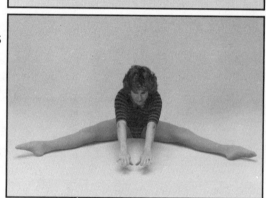

3 Bend to the right, then return to starting position and do a swan breath (inhale through your nose while moving your arms upward, then exhale through your mouth while bringing your arms down). *Repetitions:* Repeat the entire exercise five times.

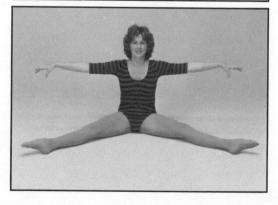

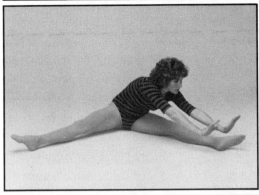

1 Lean left from your hip and stretch as far forward as you can, looking over your left foot.

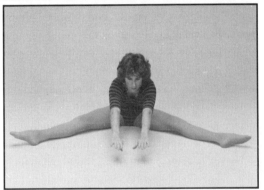

2 Bend forward at the center of your body, holding your chest as close to the floor as possible.

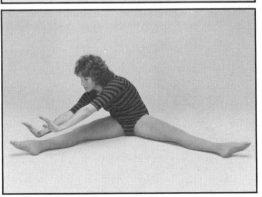

3 Bend to the right, then return to starting position and do a swan breath (inhale through your nose while moving your arms upward, then exhale through your mouth while bringing your arms down). *Repetitions:* Repeat the entire exercise five times.

Hamstring Straddle Stretch

Aim: To stretch your hamstrings and tone your legs, buttocks, arms, and shoulders.

Starting Position: Straddle sit, with your toes pointed comfortably and your arms at your sides.

Exercise No. 13

Abdominal Series

Aim: To strengthen your abdominal muscles.

Starting Positions: #1. Hook-lying, with your arms crossed, holding your ribs. #2. Hook-lying, with your arms bent and your fingers locked or hands crossed on top of your head. #3. Sit with your knees to your chest and hug your ribs, crossing your arms over your abdomen for support.

Note: If your back hurts when you do this exercise, remember to roll up slowly. Begin with starting position #1 and work up to position #2. If your abdominal muscles have separated during pregnancy, use starting position #3 to begin with.

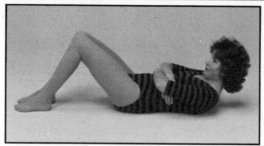

1 *Starting position #1:* Curl up, exhaling as you come up. Inhale as you curl back down to starting position. *Repetitions:* Begin with five and increase to thirty.

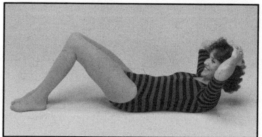

1 *Starting position #2:* Same as above, beginning in a different starting position.

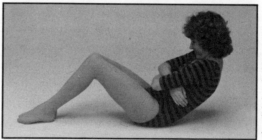

1 *Starting position #3 (diastasis variation):* Slowly curl back down to the floor, with your chin in your chest. Place one vertebra on the floor at a time.

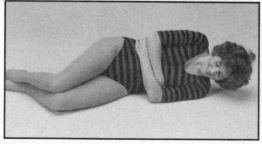

2 Roll to your left side, then return to starting position. Repeat step 1, then roll to your right side. *Repetitions:* Repeat the entire exercise ten times.

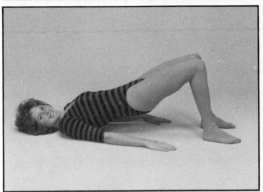

1 "Tuck" your pelvis and pull your abdominal muscles in while raising your hips slightly off the floor, resting your weight on your shoulders. Tighten your buttocks as much as you can, then release. Slowly lower your hips to the floor to starting position. *Repetitions:* Repeat five times.

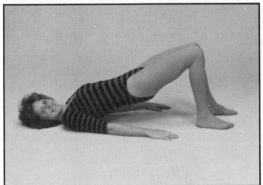

2 With your feet still apart, put your knees together, "tuck" your pelvis, and pull in your abdominal muscles. Raise your hips, then tighten and release your buttock muscles. Lower your hips to the floor to starting position. *Repetitions:* Repeat five times.

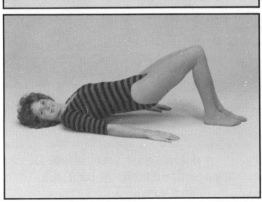

3 Put your knees and feet together and raise your hips, then tighten and release your buttock muscles. Lower your hips to the floor to starting position. *Repetitions:* Repeat five times.

Seat Squeeze

Aim: To strengthen your abdominal and buttock muscles and increase the flexibility of your back.

Starting Position: Hook-lying, with your feet slightly apart.

Note: To avoid putting pressure on your neck, do not raise your hips too high.

Back Tucks

Aim: To strengthen your abdominal muscles and stretch your lower back muscles.

Starting Position: Lying flat on your back with your arms at your sides.

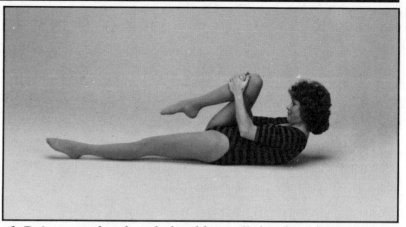

1 Raise your head and shoulders off the floor. Bring your left knee to your chest and grasp it, then bring your right knee to your chest and grasp it. Repeat five times with each leg, alternating legs.

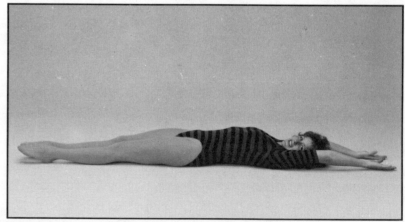

2 Return to starting position. Raise your arms above your head, point your toes, and stretch. *Repetitions:* Repeat the entire exercise two to four times.

Exercise No. 16

1 Pointing your toes, raise your left leg as high as you can, then lower it to rest on your right leg. *Repetitions:* Repeat ten times.

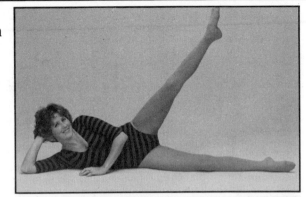

2 Keeping your toes pointed, raise your left leg slightly and circle it five times forward, then five times backward.

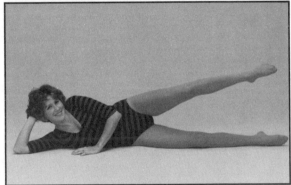

3 Raise your left leg, cross it in front of your right leg, and place it flat on the floor. Point the toes of your right foot, then straighten your right leg and lift it ten times. *Repetitions:* Repeat the entire exercise lying on your left side, with your left leg bent.

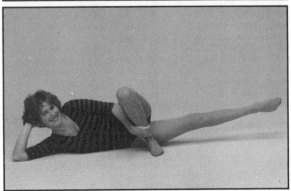

Leg Raises

Aim: To strengthen your inner and outer thighs, lower back, and buttock muscles.

Starting Position: Lying on your right side with your right knee bent, using your right arm to support your head and your left arm to steady your body.

Exercise No. 17

Rainbows
(Heel/Toe Side-Raisers)

Aim: To tone your hips, legs, waist, and buttocks.

Starting Position: Lying on your left side, using your left arm to support your head and your right arm to steady your body.

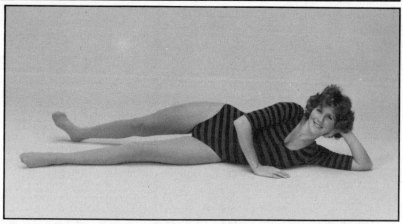

1 Bend your left leg. Raise your right leg five to eight inches off the floor, then touch your right heel down behind your left leg.

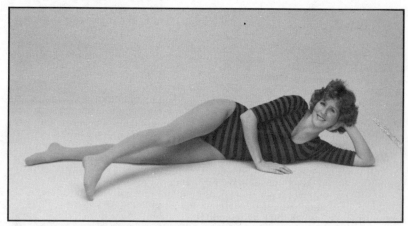

2 Bring your right foot to the front and touch your toe to the floor. Do the heel/toe motion five times, then reverse and do a toe/heel motion five times. *Repetitions:* Repeat the entire exercise lying on your right side.

1 Raise your head and shoulders off the floor. Draw your knees toward your chest until your back is off the floor and your body is in a V position.

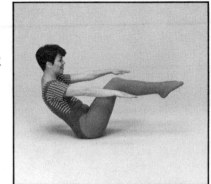

2 Keeping your arms straight in front of you, raise and lower your legs and shoulders at the same time, without touching either to the floor. *Repetitions:* Repeat ten times, working up to two sets of ten.

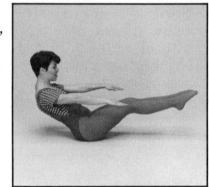

Sitting Tucks

Aim: To tighten your abdominal muscles and tone your entire body.

Starting Position: Lying on your back with your legs straight out.

1 *Tuck-sit variation:* Begin in a pike sit, with your hands on the floor, behind your hips, and your arms slightly bent. Keeping your arms bent, tuck your knees toward your chest.

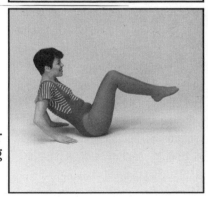

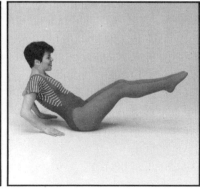

2 Extend both legs, bending your elbows slightly for balance. Keep your hips on the floor and your knees slightly bent as you extend your legs. Tuck and extend your legs without letting your feet touch the floor. *Repetitions:* Do one or two sets of ten tucks.

Exercise No. 19

Hamstring Stretch

Aim: To stretch your hamstring muscles and strengthen your leg and buttock muscles.

Starting Position: Standing with your feet together and your knees slightly relaxed.

Note: Keep your knees relaxed throughout the exercise.

1 Clasp your hands behind your back.

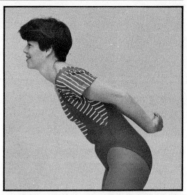

2 Keeping your head up, bend forward from the hips until you feel a stretch at the backs of your legs. Hold this position for five seconds.

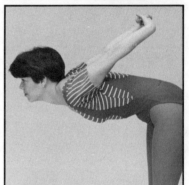

3 Bend your knees, round your back, drop your chin to your chest, and release your hands. Slowly straighten up. Reach tall with your head and stand straight, then tighten your abdominal muscles and shake your shoulders slightly. *Repetitions:* Repeat the entire exercise five times.

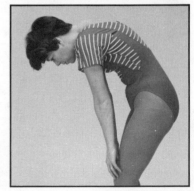

1 *Arm Circles:* With your palms up, move your arms forward to make five to ten small circles, then five to ten large circles. *Repetitions:* Repeat moving your arms backward, then repeat with your palms down.

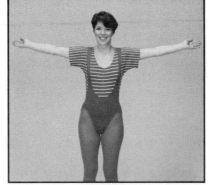

1 *Wrist Flexors:* Moving only your wrists, point your fingertips toward the ceiling, then toward the floor. *Repetitions:* Repeat five to ten times.

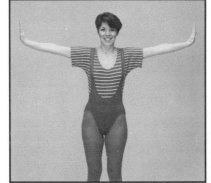

Arm Series

Aim: To strengthen your upper and lower arms, wrists, and pectoral muscles.

Starting Position: Standing with your feet shoulders'-width apart and your arms in cross position.

1 *Scarecrow:* With your palms facing backward, spread your fingers. Keeping your upper arms at shoulder height, bend your arms at the elbows and swing your arms in front of your body, then return to starting position. *Repetitions:* Repeat five to ten times.

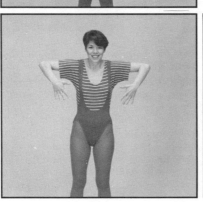

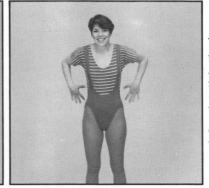

1 *Back Sweeper:* With your palms facing backward, bend your arms at the elbows and try to bring your fingertips together behind your back, then return to starting position. *Repetitions:* Repeat five to ten times slowly.

Exercise No. 20

Arm Series

Aim: To strengthen your upper and lower arms, wrists, and pectoral muscles.

Starting Position: Standing with your feet shoulders'-width apart and your arms in cross position.

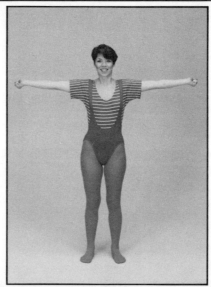

1 *Elbow Flex:* With your palms up, make fists. Bring your fists to your shoulders, then continue to move them downward and outward in an arc.

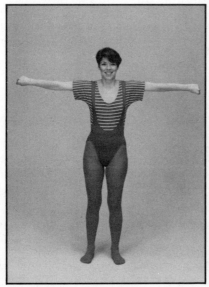

2 With your hands still fisted, turn your wrists toward the ceiling.

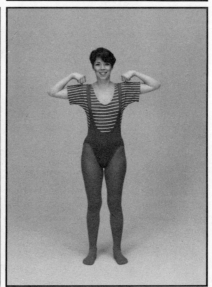

3 Bend your elbows and touch your fists to your shoulders, then return to starting position. *Repetitions:* Repeat five to ten times.

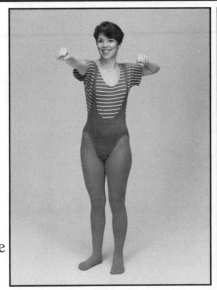

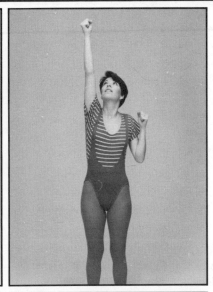

1 *Arm Punches:* Make fists. Punch forward five to ten times, alternating arms.

2 Punch over your head five to ten times, alternating arms.

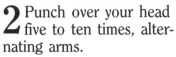

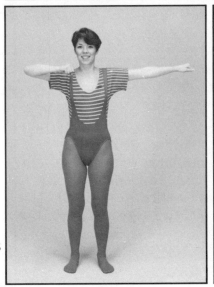

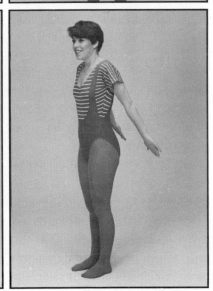

3 Punch out to your sides five to ten times, alternating arms.

1 *Push Backs:* Turn your palms toward your back and gently press up and back. *Repetitions:* Repeat five to ten times.

Exercise No. 21

Leg Lifts

Aim: To tone your leg muscles.

Starting Position: Standing at a wall, with your palms resting comfortably against the wall, or standing beside a chair, with the palm of your left hand on the back of the chair.

1 Draw your right knee into your chest and relax your left knee, keeping your back straight. Circle your right foot five times in each direction.

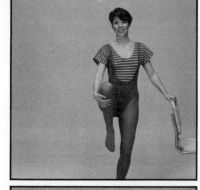

2 Keeping your left knee slightly bent, draw your right knee to your right side.

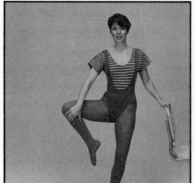

3 Drop your right leg to a comfortable position and straighten it. Bend and straighten your right leg ten times. *Repetitions:* Repeat the entire exercise with your left leg.

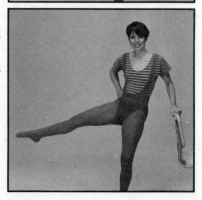

Exercise No. 22

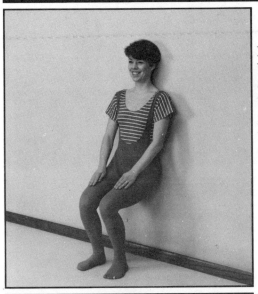

1 Bend your knees and slide your upper body down. "Sit" with your thighs at a right angle to the wall, as if you were sitting on a stool. Press the small of your back firmly against the wall. (This is a great time to practice kegels.) Hold the position for twenty to forty-five seconds.

Skier's Sit

Aim: To strengthen your legs, abdominal muscles, and lower back.

Starting Position: Standing with your back against a wall.

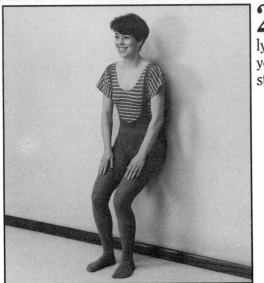

2 Lean forward and place your hands on your knees, then slowly straighten your back. Straighten your knees slowly and return to a standing position.

Exercise No. 23

Calf Stretch

Aim: To stretch your calf muscles in preparation for walking.

Starting Position: Standing with your hands on the wall, your toes pointed forward, and your hips pressed forward.

1 Put your right foot forward with your knee bent, and stretch your left leg behind you (keep both heels on the floor). Keeping your lower back flat, hold a comfortable stretch for fifteen seconds. Do not bounce. *Repetitions:* Repeat with your left foot forward.

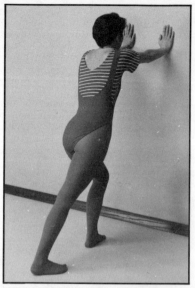

2 *Variation:* As you stretch, lean forward and rest your head on your hands.

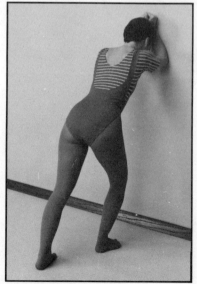

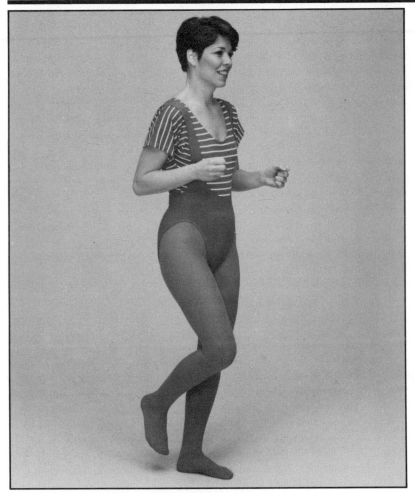

Walking/ Jogging

Aim: To strengthen your cardiovascular system and your legs.

1 Walk briskly or jog. Strive for fifteen to twenty minutes with your heart rate between fifty and seventy percent of your maximum target heart rate. (See pages 8 to 10 for information about the cardiovascular system and target heart rate.)

113

Exercise No. 24

Side Lean

Aim: To trim your waistline.

Starting Position: Standing two or three feet from a wall (or a partner), with your left arm at shoulder height and your left palm against the wall.

1 Extend your right arm overhead with your left elbow locked, and stretch toward the wall. Reach over your head with your right arm, pushing your hips out as you do so. Try to touch your right hand to the wall.

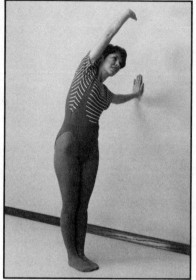

2 As you bring your right arm down, press your hips toward the wall (be sure to keep your left elbow locked). *Repetitions:* Repeat the entire exercise three to five times on your left side, then repeat three to five times with your right palm against the wall.

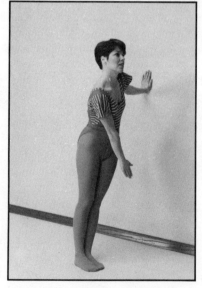

1 *Side-to-side sway:* Sway from side to side, keeping your hips and shoulders in vertical alignment. *Repetitions:* Repeat five times.

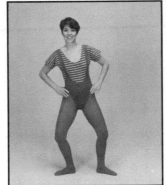

Plié Series

2 *Stride sway:* Keeping your feet shoulders'-width apart, take one step forward with your left foot. Sway forward and back, keeping your heels on the floor. *Repetitions:* Repeat ten times with each foot, then return to starting position and repeat the *side-to-side sway* five times.

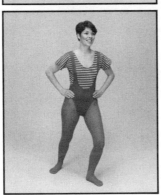

Aim: To tone your legs, waist, buttock muscles, and lower back.

Starting Position: Standing with your feet shoulders'-width apart, with your pelvis tucked, your abdominal muscles pulled in, your knees flexed, and your toes and knees aligned.

3 *Elbow-hip sway:* Place your hands on your shoulders and lower your right elbow to your right hip, then return to upright position. Lower your left elbow to your left hip, then return to upright position. *Repetitions:* Repeat ten times, alternating sides. Return to starting position and repeat the *side-to-side sway* five times.

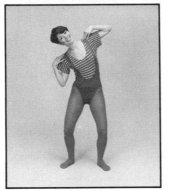

Exercise No. 26

Bicycles on Elbows

Aim: To strengthen your abdomen and lower back muscles, and to increase the circulation in and mobility of your legs.

Starting Position: Lying on your back, supporting your upper-body weight on your elbows.

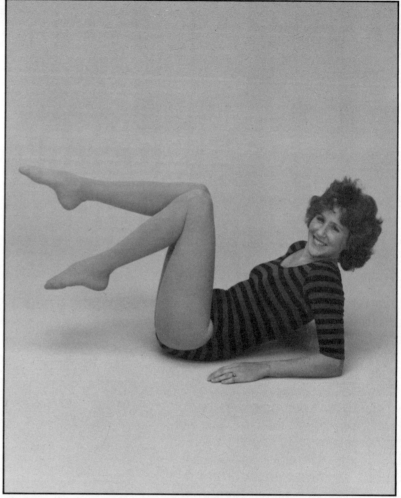

Note: This is a fun exercise to do side-by-side with your baby because the baby will try to imitate your movements.

1 Bicycle forward and reverse for thirty seconds. Rest, then bicycle another thirty seconds. *Repetitions:* Work up to a full five to ten minutes of bicycling (a kitchen timer may be helpful).

116

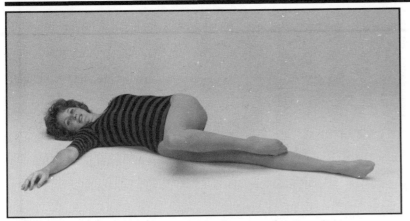

1 Draw your left knee to your chest and cross it over your body. Hold the position for five seconds.

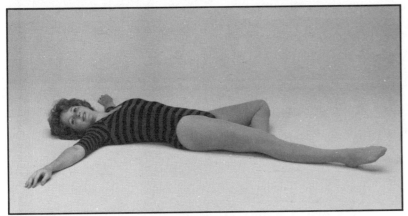

2 Place the instep of your left foot on the inside of your right knee. Hold your left knee as close to the floor as is comfortable, until you feel a stretch. Hold the position for five seconds, then relax. *Repetitions:* Repeat the entire exercise three to five times with each leg, alternating legs.

Knee Cross-Overs

Aim: To stretch your lower back muscles and tone your buttock muscles.

Starting Position: Lying on your back with your legs straight out.

Exercise No. 28

Leg Circles

Aim: To tone your legs and buttocks.

Starting Position: All fours.

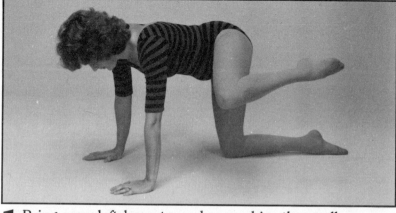

1 Bring your left knee toward your chin, then roll your left hip to the side. Open your leg out so that the inner thigh of your left leg is parallel to the floor.

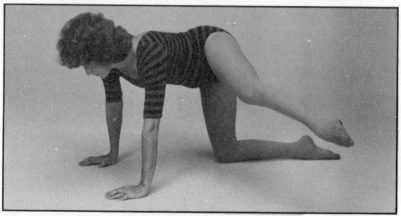

2 Straighten your left leg, keeping your knee parallel to the floor. Look straight down at the floor as you circle your leg forward twice with your foot flexed, then twice with your toes pointed. *Repetitions:* Repeat twice with each leg, alternating sides; work up to four or more times with each leg.

Note: To make this exercise really work for you, tighten your buttocks while you circle your legs.

118

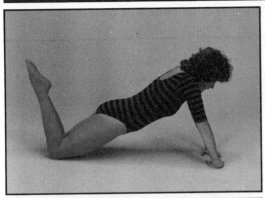

1 Bend your knees and push up, exhaling as you do so.

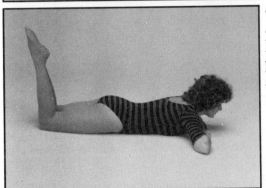

2 Inhale as you slowly lower yourself toward the floor. *Repetitions:* Repeat five times. Add two or three push-ups each week as you gain strength; work up to twenty or more.

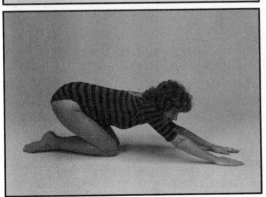

1 *Let-Downs (variation for beginners):* Beginning in push-up position with your knees bent, slowly lower your body to the floor. Push your body back so that your hips are aligned with your heels, then return to starting position. *Repetitions:* Repeat three to five times; work up to ten let-downs.

Push-Ups

Aim: To strengthen your shoulders and your pectoral muscles.

Starting Position: Lying flat on your stomach, with your hands under your shoulders and your fingers pointed in.

Note: To make the push-ups more difficult, bring your fingertips closer together. Beginners should start with the *Let-down* variation.

Exercise No. 30

Cheek to Cheek

Aim: To tone your buttock muscles.

Starting Position: Lying flat on your stomach, with your forehead resting on your folded forearms.

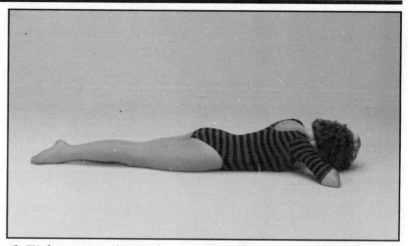

1 Tighten your buttock muscles. Hold the position for fifteen seconds, then release. *Repetitions:* Repeat three to five times.

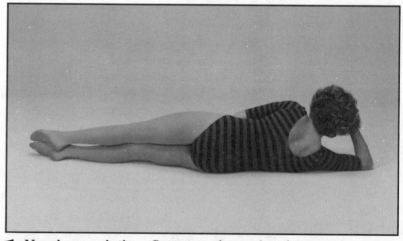

1 *Nursing variation:* Same as above, but lying on your side.

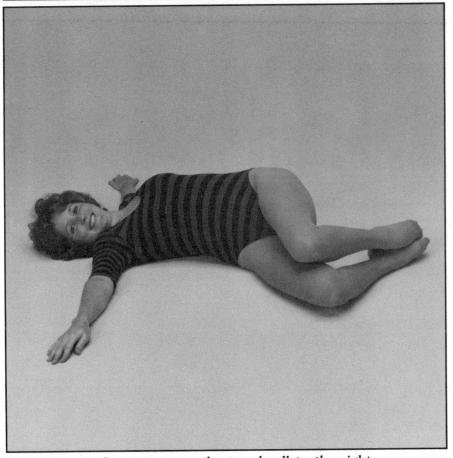

Hip Roll

Aim: To trim your hips, waist, and thighs.

Starting Position: Hook-lying, with your arms in cross position.

1 Bring your knees to your chest and roll to the right. Bring your knees back to center, then roll to the left. *Repetitions:* Repeat ten times on each side, alternating sides.

Exercise No. 32

V-Stretch

Aim: To tone and strengthen your abdominal muscles, legs, feet, and especially your inner thighs.

Starting Position: Back tuck.

1 Open your knees wide, place your toes together, and slide your hands down to your ankles.

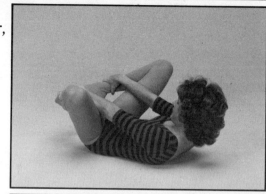

2 Pull your feet close to your body, then slowly straighten your legs out to a V position. Hold the position for a few seconds. Do not bounce.

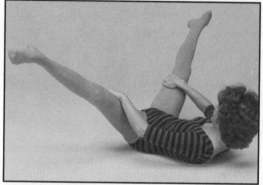

3 Keeping your knees open wide, bring your toes back together, then return to starting position. *Repetitions:* Repeat five times.

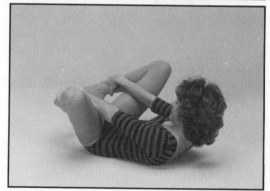

1 Slowly roll to the right.

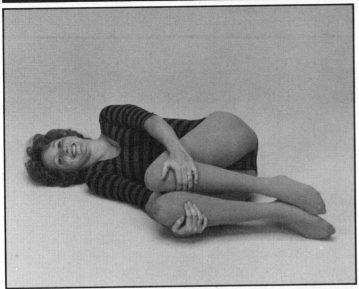

Lower Back Roll

Aim: To massage your lower back and stretch your inner thighs.

Starting Position: Back tuck.

2 Open your legs far enough to feel a stretch in your inner thighs and to create the need to roll to the left, then do so. *Repetitions:* Roll from side to side three to five times (the rolling motion will massage your lower back).

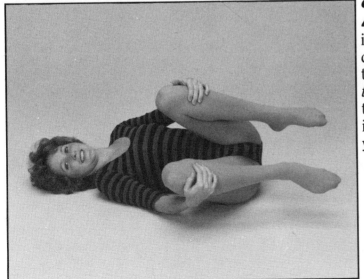

Exercise No. 34

Knee Gliders

Aim: To relax your lower back, hips, and buttock muscles.

Starting Position: Lying on your left side with your head resting comfortably on your arm, and with your hips and knees slightly bent.

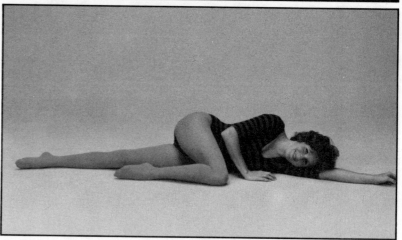

1 Bring your right knee over your left side, shifting your weight to your right hip as you do so.

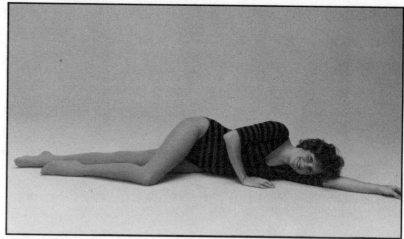

2 Keeping your right knee on the floor, glide it toward your chest and back down until your leg is almost straight. *Repetitions:* Repeat three times on each side.

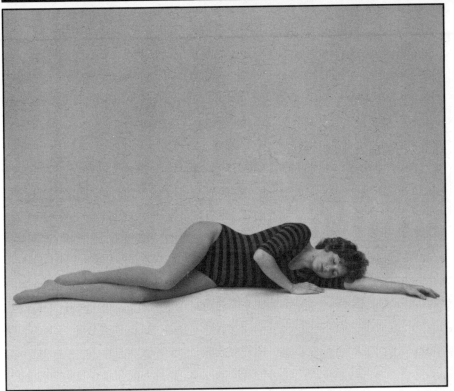

Body Relaxation

Aim: To relax you.

Starting Position: Lying on your left side.

1 Concentrate on something or somewhere very peaceful. Close your eyes and take deep breaths. In the following order, relax your *feet, legs, back, arms, neck, and face*. After you feel totally relaxed and peaceful, open your eyes, roll to all fours, and slowly stand up.

Exercise No. 36

Leg Elevations

Aim: To improve the circulation in your legs.

Starting Position: Lying flat on your back with your feet flat against a wall or resting on a chair.

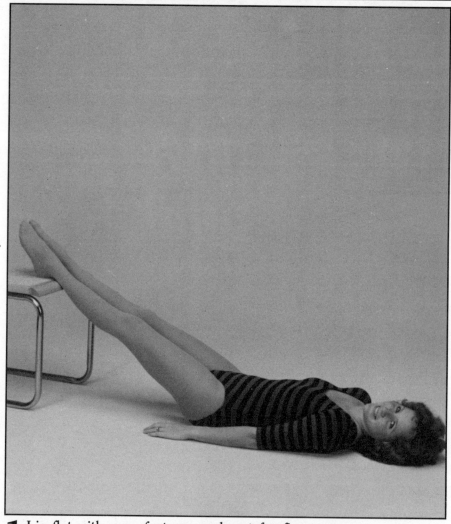

Note: Your legs need to be elevated only above your heart.

1 Lie flat with your feet up, and rest for five to ten minutes. Roll to your side, sit for a moment to prevent light-headedness, then stand up.

Chapter Four
Focus on the Baby

Baby exercises? Yes! You can begin exercising with your baby right from the start. This chapter includes a section on massages for your baby, a description of your baby's reflexes that can be "patterned" through exercise to help your baby develop coordination and motor skills, and two sets of parent/baby exercises— one for newborn to four-month-old babies, the other for four- to twelve-month-old babies. At the end of this chapter are directions for making your own exercise equipment (an exercise mat/roll and a beanbag chair).

These parent/baby exercises give you a time to play meaningfully with your child and encourage self-discovery and the development of physical control in your baby. These activities also begin to establish movement patterns, stimulate your baby's circulation, and help his or her muscular development. In addition, parent/baby exercise helps your child become aware early on that daily exercise is a vital part of health.

These exercises follow the natural sequence of motor skill development, providing the fundamentals for sitting, crawling, and walking. While there is no guarantee that a child who does the exercises will walk earlier or recognize you sooner than a child who does not, the exercises will help you guide and encourage your child's motor development.

Suggestions for Exercising Your Baby

When should you exercise your baby? With babies, it is not important that you set aside a certain time of day to do an exercise routine. Rather, you should fit the exercise techniques into your baby's everyday activities. For example:

• Start the baby's day with a stimulating massage, followed by some stretching exercises.

• After a bath or prior to naptime, try one of the relaxation exercises or relaxing massages.

• After naptime, work on patterning and exercises related to developing the baby's motor skills.

• Before bedtime, practice relaxation exercises, followed by a relaxing massage.

For older babies, continue to use massage or relaxation techniques that include a range of motion for the joints. Add two or three exercises at a time, depending on your baby's muscle strength and motor skill level. The Family Team Exercises on pages 162 to 176 will provide exercise both for you and your baby. There are even some exercises for mom, dad, and baby to do as a family.

• Exercise on a soft, warm, secure surface.
• Make your baby feel secure by supporting him or her properly.
• Don't overtire your baby. A reasonable amount of time for a newborn is five minutes.
• Don't ever strain or put pressure on the baby.
• Don't exercise body joints after eating.
• Exercise with your baby for short periods of time, several times a day.
• Increase the length of exercise time as the baby gets older.
• Always move body parts through natural motions (i.e., no side movement of knees).
• Relax and have fun. Exercise is a time to be enjoyed by both parents and child.

Do's and Don'ts for Exercising Your Baby

Baby Massage

Massage provides a unique way to relate to your baby, while offering him a number of benefits: it maintains his levels of activity and movement, stimulates his sense of touch, helps him relax, tones his muscles, and can stimulate his organic and psychological growth. At the same time, massage enhances your feelings of competence in being able to handle your child. Most of all, baby massage gives you a special time together each day. Practice the three massages on pages 128 to 130 to help you get started with a regular baby massage routine.

Basic Directions

• Choose a warm place (e.g., the side of a pool or a bathtub) for a massage, and be sure your hands are warm.

• Use firm but gentle strokes.

• Maintain hand and eye contact with your baby throughout the massage, and don't lift your hands off and on the baby.

• Talk to your baby. Let your touch tell him how much you love him.

Vocabulary

Milk—with a light squeeze, move your hands "toward the heart" for circulation benefits. Work on one area at a time—for example, when massaging the baby's arm, milk from his hand to his shoulder. For a relaxing massage, milk "outward from the heat," i.e., move from the warmer to cooler areas of the body.

Comb—with your hand open and fingers spread, try for a lighter touch with each combing action (watch your nails to avoid scratching the baby).

Rake—a milking motion, using alternate sides of your hands.

Stimulating Massage

Note: This massage is best used prior to exercising. Don't do it right before nap- or bedtime, as it will tend to stimulate your baby.

Starting Position: Lay your baby on her back on a firm, comfortable surface.

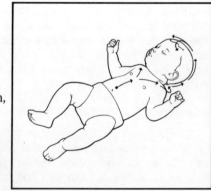

1 Using a small circular motion, massage, in the following order: a) her stomach; b) her chest; c) her shoulders; d) the back of her neck; e) the back of her head; f) the top of her head; g) her temples.

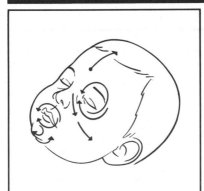

2 Using a slight sweeping motion with your thumb, massage: a) her forehead, from center to hairline; b) around her eyes—circle one way, then the other; c) the sides of her nose—sweep down and across to her cheeks; d) her cheeks—stroke from her chin diagonally to her hairline; e) her mouth—circle your finger around her lips one way, then the other; f) her chin—circle your finger around her chin one way, then the other.

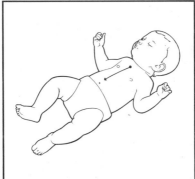

3 Using small, circular motions, massage her chest; then rake her abdominal area.

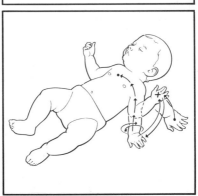

4 Massage her left arm, then: a) stroke the back of her left hand and palm, then separate her fingers; b) gently shake and squeeze her left hand; c) using a range of motion, bend her left elbow, straighten it, then circle her left arm, rotating it in and out; d) milk her left arm gently and massage her chest. Repeat step 4 with her right arm.

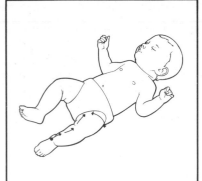

5 Using a circular motion, massage your baby's trunk down her left leg, then: a) using a milking stroke, massage her left leg; b) flex her left hip and circle it in a range of motion; c) flex her left knee and rotate her hip in and out.

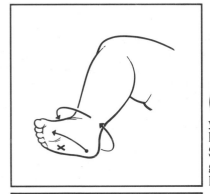

6 Circle her left ankle and separate her toes. Then, using your thumbs, massage the sole of her left foot from heel to toes. Shake her left foot and squeeze it gently. Repeat steps 5 and 6 with her right leg.

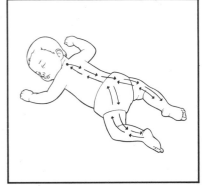

7 Turn your baby onto her stomach (if she won't lie on her stomach, try placing her stomach across your legs), then: a) using your cupped hand, massage your baby starting at her neck, then moving your hand down to her buttocks, and then to her heel; b) comb her back with your fingers (watch out for your fingernails).

Relaxing Massage

Note: Best used prior to bedtime or naptime, or with a fussy baby.

Starting Position: Lay your baby on his back or across your lap.

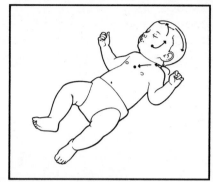 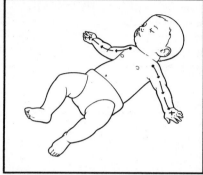 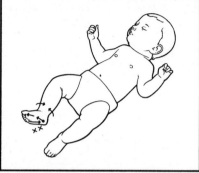

1 Using small, circular motions with your fingers, massage around your baby's face and head, over his shoulders, and on his chest.

2 Milk his left arm outward, then shake and gently squeeze his left hand. Repeat with his right arm.

3 Using small, circular motions with your fingers, massage your baby's trunk down his left leg. Then: a) roll his left leg between your hands; and b) with your thumbs, massage the sole of his left foot from heel to toes. Repeat steps with his right leg. Shake the baby's legs, then comb his chest and squeeze each of his feet twice.

Simple Back Massage

Starting Position: Lay your baby face down on a soft towel or on your lap.

1 Using small, circular motions, massage your baby, starting at the back of her neck. a) Go down her shoulders to her arms, then squeeze her hands gently; b) go down her back, buttocks, and legs; c) gently squeeze her calves and feet; d) go up her legs, buttocks, and back to the back of her neck; e) comb her back.

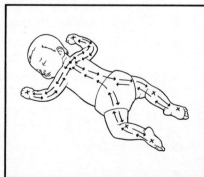

Patterning Your Baby's Reflexes

Infants can make very few voluntary movements other than a few with their arms and legs. Most of the movements they do make are reflexive—i.e., automatic reactions to stimulation. As infants repeat these movements over and over, they begin to develop patterns that become the basis for voluntary movements later. Stimulating these movements through the use of exercises you can do with your baby can help him or her develop appropriate patterns.

This type of patterning can be done with babies in a way that allows a joint to move through a specific range of movement while coordinating with the movement of another joint. While this process does not assure earlier completion of any specific motor skill such as crawling or walking, it may aid your baby when his or her perception and physical maturity are developed.

"Patterning" exercises can be used from birth. Chart 4a lists six common reflexes of newborns and four voluntary reflexes that appear later, together with exercises that test the reflexes.

Chart 4a.   Exercises for Patterning Your Baby's Reflexes

Name of Reflex	Description	Exercise(s)
1. Stepping	If your baby is placed in a standing position on his feet, he will respond by stepping.	
2. Palmar grasp	Your baby's hand will curl tightly around any object placed in it.	Baby Pull-ups, page 140.
3. Babinski reflex	If you stroke the sole of your baby's foot, her toes will fan out and her big toe will extend.	Relaxation and Foot Toner, page 132.
4. Righting reflex (China doll reflex)	If you hold your baby upright, he will try to keep his head up and his eyes open.	Neck Strength Test, page 145.
5. Tonic neck reflex (fencer position)	When a baby turns her head to one side, with one arm at her side, and extends that arm, the opposite arm flexes. This reflex may help her use the sides of her body separately.	Roll to Side, page 143.
6. Swimming reflex	When a baby is placed in water, he makes swimming motions.	Frog Kick and Whip Kick, page 139.
7. Reciprocal kicking	If you hold your baby straight out in front of you, she will kick her legs alternately. This reflex usually disappears after the first month.	Bicycles, Bicycle Flutters, and Bicycle Scissors, page 141.
8. Neck righting	If your baby's head is turned, his body will follow. This reflex appears when the tonic neck reflex disappears.	Rock 'n' Roll, page 144.
9. Parachute reflex (supporting reflex)	If your baby begins to fall forward from an upright position, she will try to catch herself.	Games on the Roll, pages 156 and 157.
10. Landau reflex	If a baby is held under his stomach only, he will extend his arms and legs. This reflex indicates back strength.	Sky Diver/Parachute, page 164.

Exercise No. 1

Relaxation

Aim: To relax your baby's body and tone his feet.

Starting Position: Lay your baby on his back.

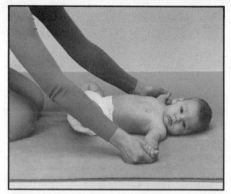

1 Bring his hands together, then slowly lower his arms to cross position.

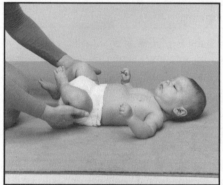

2 Place an index finger under each knee and toss his legs up and down lightly, then bring his knees close to his chest, one at a time. Move his knees only as far as they can easily go—never push or force them.

1 *Foot Toner:* Place a finger in the instep of your baby's left foot and place your thumb on the ball of his left foot. Flex his left foot, pointing his toes ten times slowly. Circle his left foot ten times slowly to the left, then ten times to the right. *Repetitions:* Repeat with his right foot.

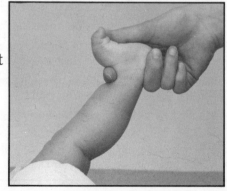

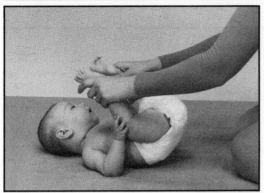

1 Holding your baby's ankles, slowly bring her feet over her head toward the floor. Allow her legs to come back down slowly. *Repetitions:* Repeat five times.

Diaper Change

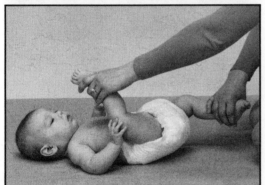

1 *Variation:* With your baby in the same starting position, raise her left hand above her head and raise her right foot toward her hand. Repeat five times on each side, alternating sides.

Aim: To promote flexibility in your baby's back and help relieve gas (especially helpful with colicky babies).

Starting Position: Lay your baby on her back.

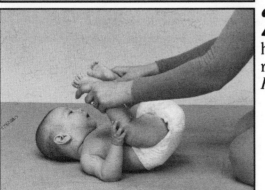

2 Bring both feet over the top of her head and hold for two seconds, then return to starting position. *Repetitions:* Repeat once.

Note: Make a game of this exercise by peeking through your baby's legs while they are over her head.

Exercise No. 3

Hug and Rock

Aim: Stretches your baby's arms and promotes his body awareness; may help calm a crying baby.

Starting Position: Lay your baby on his back and cross his arms over his abdomen.

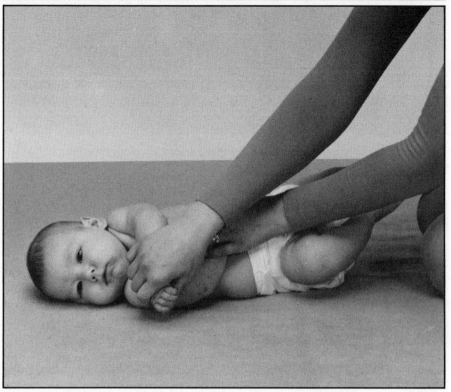

1 Grip your baby's forearms and let him hug himself and touch the rest of his body. Rock him gently to the right and left.

Exercise No. 4

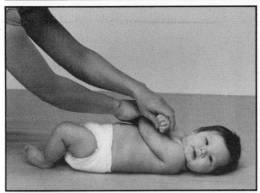

1 Holding your baby's hands, cross her left arm over her right arm, then cross her right arm over her left arm. *Repetitions:* Repeat three to five times with each arm, alternating arms.

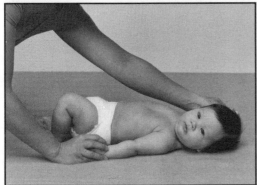

2 Raise her left arm above her head, then lower it. Raise her right arm above her head and lower it. *Repetitions:* Repeat three to five times with each arm, alternating arms.

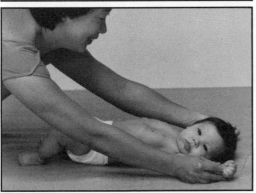

3 Holding your baby's wrists, slowly stretch her arms in a V above her head, then lower her arms.

Arm Stretching

Aim: To stretch your baby's arms; a good warm-up exercise.

Starting Position: Lay your baby on her back.

Note: To promote your baby's self-esteem, say "yeah" each time you stretch her limbs in the V position, and clap when you finish the exercise.

135

Exercise No. 4

Leg Stretching

Aim: To stretch your baby's legs; a good warm-up exercise.

Starting Position: Lay your baby on her back.

1 Holding your baby's ankles, cross her left leg over her right leg, then cross her right leg over her left leg. *Repetitions:* Repeat three to five times with each leg, alternating legs.

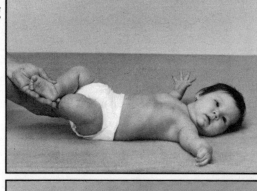

2 Raise her left leg above her head, then lower it. Raise her right leg above her head, then lower it. *Repetitions:* Repeat three to five times with each leg, alternating legs.

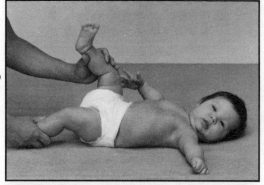

3 Holding onto your baby's ankles, slowly stretch her legs into a V position.

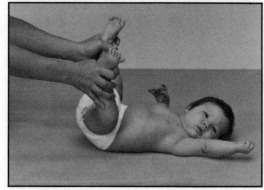

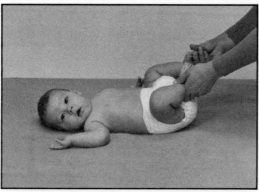

1 Bend your baby's knees, bringing them up to his chest.

Flex and Extend

Aim: To strengthen your baby's thigh muscles and help relieve gas pains.

Starting Position: Lay your baby on his back and hold onto his ankles.

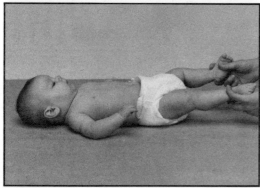

2 Slowly straighten his legs. Be sure your baby's legs are off the floor slightly; never straighten his legs and press them flat to the ground. *Repetitions:* Repeat three to five times.

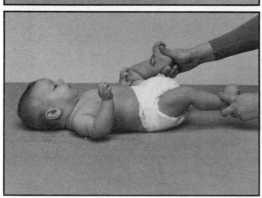

1 *Variation:* Alternate bringing his left and right knees to his chest five times, alternating legs.

Note: If your baby resists, squeeze his feet and encourage him to relax.

137

Exercise No. 6

1 Cross your baby's right arm and left leg at her middle.

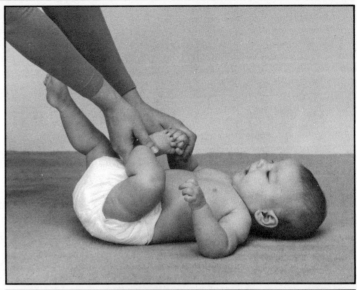

Criss-Cross

Aim: To stretch your baby's arms, legs, and back.

Starting Position: Lay your baby on her back and hold onto her right wrist and left ankle.

2 Stretch her limbs in opposite directions, then return to starting position. Cross and stretch her left arm and right leg. *Repetitions:* Repeat three to five times on each side, alternating sides.

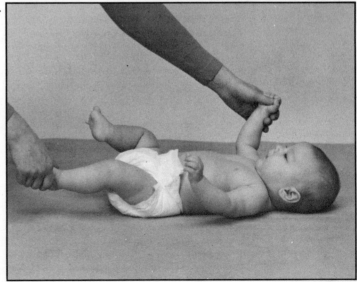

1 *Frog Kick:* Holding onto your baby's ankles, bend his knees to his chest.

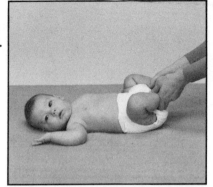

Exercise No. 7

Kicks

2 With his legs slightly off the floor, straighten his legs into a V, then bring his legs back together and bend his knees to his chest. *Repetitions:* Repeat five times.

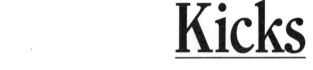

Aim: To tone your baby's leg muscles.

Starting Position: *Frog Kick:* Lay your baby on his back. *Whip Kick:* Lay your baby on his stomach.

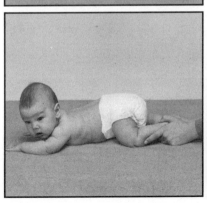

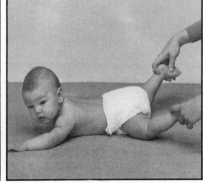

1 *Whip Kick:* Hold your baby's ankles and bend his knees, tucking them underneath him.

2 Gliding his legs along the floor, move his legs down and outward, then back together. Bend his knees and tuck his legs back under him. *Repetitions:* Repeat five times.

139

Exercise No. 8

Pull-Ups

Aim: To strengthen your baby's chest, hands and arms.

Starting Position: *Monkey Grip* and *Pull-ups:* Lay your baby on her back. *See-saws:* Pike sit.

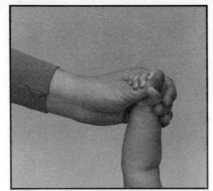

1 *Monkey Grip:* Have your baby grasp your thumbs with both hands (Palmar grasp); wrap your index finger around her hands to be sure she holds her grip.

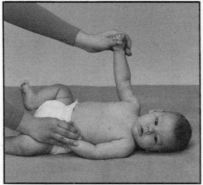

2 Gently pull one arm at a time in an easy upward motion. Do not lift her from the surface, although one shoulder may rise slightly. *Repetitions:* Repeat two or three times with each arm.

1 *Pull-ups:* Repeat step 1 above, then gently pull *both* arms upward until she just begins to lift off the floor. Keeping your hands very still, allow your baby to pull herself up to your fingers. *Repetitions:* Repeat two or three times.

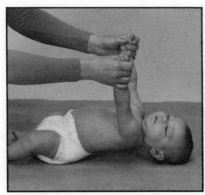

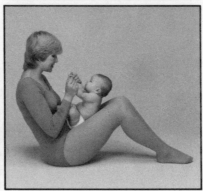

1 *See-saws (sit-ups for babies two to four months old):* Bend your knees and place your baby on your stomach with her facing you, her back against your thighs. Hold her hands as you do sit-ups with her resting on your thighs. *Repetitions:* Repeat five to ten times.

140

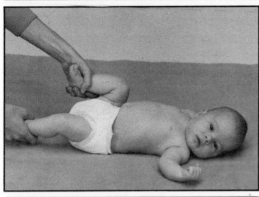

1 Place your hands under his knees and pedal his legs in an up-and-down motion for twenty seconds. Lift his hips off the floor slightly and pedal his legs for another twenty seconds.

Exercise No. 9

Bicycles

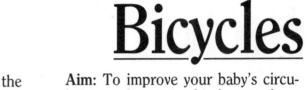

1 *Flutters:* With your baby in the same starting position, hold onto his feet. Extend his legs and lift them off the floor slightly. Make small, light kicking movements (flutters) with the baby's feet for twenty seconds.

Aim: To improve your baby's circulation and exercise his legs at the hip socket.

Starting Position: Lay your baby on his back.

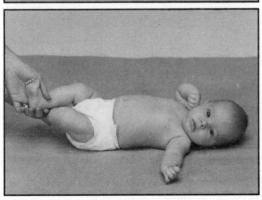

1 *Scissors:* With your baby in the same starting position, hold his legs straight out in front of him, parallel to the floor. Scissor his left leg past his right leg so that his legs just touch. Scissor his right leg past his left leg. *Repetitions:* Repeat ten times, alternating legs.

Note: Never force or push your baby's movements.

141

Exercise No. 10

Neck Strengtheners

Aim: To strengthen your baby's neck in preparation for crawling.

Starting Position: *Find Me:* Lay your baby on her stomach, with her face turned to her right side. *Look at Me* and *Raising Up:* Sit on the floor and lay your baby on her stomach, with her head resting against your chest.

Note: Before doing *Look at Me,* your baby must be able to turn her head. Before doing *Raising Up,* your baby should be able to lift her head or hold it up. As she gets better at *Raising Up,* have her lie on the towel on an exercise mat instead of on your chest.

1 *Find Me:* Go to your baby's left side and call her name. When she moves her head to her left side, smile at her or hand her a favorite toy. Go to her right side and call her name. *Repetitions:* Repeat *no more than* two times to each side.

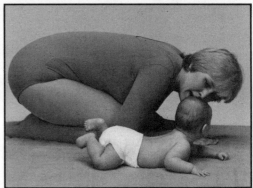

1 *Look at Me:* Lean back until you are resting on your elbows. Talk to your baby; she will lift her head. Do not make her hold her head up longer than ten seconds; then let her rest. Increase the duration as your baby's neck gets stronger.

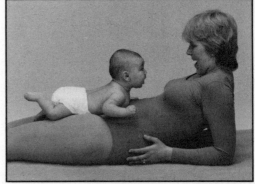

1 *Raising Up:* Same as *Look at Me,* but place a rolled-up towel under your baby's stomach and chest. *Repetitions:* Let your baby hold her head up no longer than ten seconds to start.

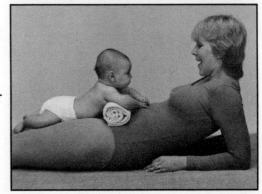

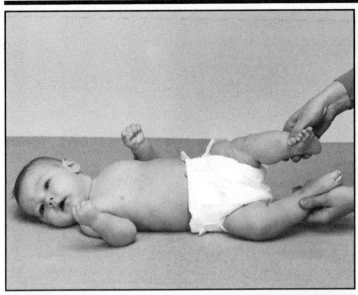

1 Raise your baby's right arm alongside his head. Hold him under his left knee, bend his knee toward his chest, and lift his seat slightly.

Exercise No. 11

Roll to Side

Aim: To prepare your baby to roll over.

Starting Position: Lay your baby on his back and place a toy about six inches away from his head.

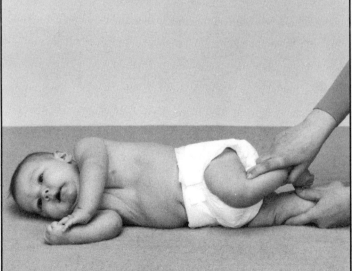

2 Roll him slowly onto his right side. *Repetitions:* Repeat, rolling him to his left side, holding his left knee.

Note: You can practice this exercise twice a day, but no more than three or four times per session.

143

Exercise No. 12

Rock 'n' Roll

Aim: To teach your baby to roll from his back to his stomach.

Starting Position: Lay your baby on her back.

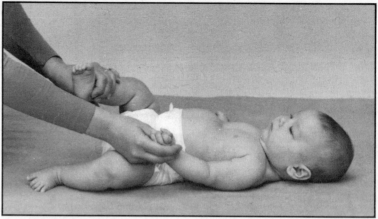

1 Bend your baby's left arm and place it on her chest. Flex her right hip, then roll her body to the left.

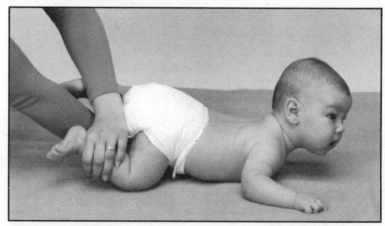

2 She will end up on her stomach. Allow her to try to free her arm, but help her if it appears to be too much of a struggle. *Repetitions:* Repeat two times to the left, then place her right arm across her chest and repeat two times to the right.

Note: Before attempting this exercise, be sure your baby has mastered rolling to her side.

1 Place one arm across your baby's chest, and the other across his hips.

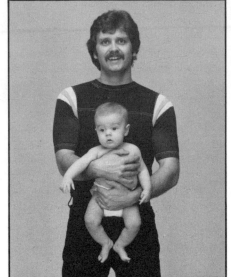

Exercises 13 through 25 (pages 145 to 161) are for babies between four and twelve months old. For exercises that benefit both you and your baby, see the Family Team Exercises on pages 162 to 176.

Strength Test

2 Slide your arm down from his chest, then look to see whether his head drops. If he is not holding his head up, wait two or three weeks before trying the exercises that follow; work on exercise #10, *Neck Strengtheners* (page 142).

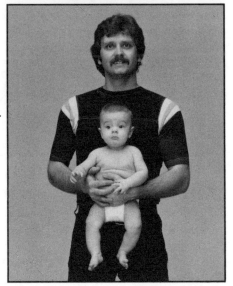

Aim: To test your baby's neck muscles to see if he is ready for some of the exercises that follow.

Starting Position: Stand, holding your baby with his back against your chest.

Note: Use this exercise to determine whether or not you should proceed with exercises that require your baby to hold his head up.

Exercise No. 14

Flagpole

Aim: To strengthen your baby's lower back.

Starting Position: Stand, holding your baby with her back against your chest, with your arms across her pelvic area.

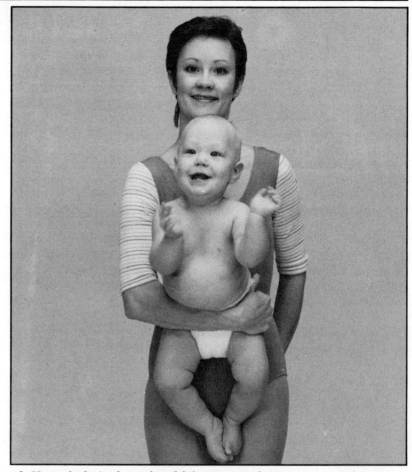

1 Your baby's feet should be pressed into your abdomen. Hold this position for a few seconds. Practice carrying your baby around the house in this position. In this carrying position, the baby's weight is at your midline, which is good for your posture; and she can see out windows and look in mirrors.

Note: Use the *Strength Test* on page 145 to see whether your baby is ready for this exercise.

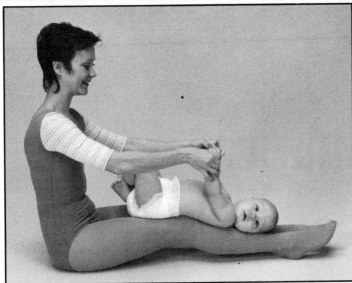

1 Gently raise your knees so that your baby's back arches slightly. Move slowly and don't raise your knees too high.

Exercise No. 15

Back Arch

Aim: To strengthen your baby's abdominal muscles.

Starting Position: Pike sit. Lay your baby on his back on your lap, with his head pointing toward your feet.

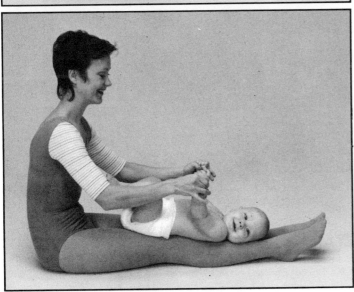

2 Return to starting position. *Repetitions:* Repeat three to five times.

Exercise No. 16

Diaper Change

Aim: To promote flexibility in your baby's back and help relieve gas (especially helpful with colicky babies).

Starting Position: Lay your baby on her back.

1 Holding your baby's ankles, slowly bring her feet over her head toward the floor. Allow her legs to come back down slowly. *Repetitions:* Repeat five times.

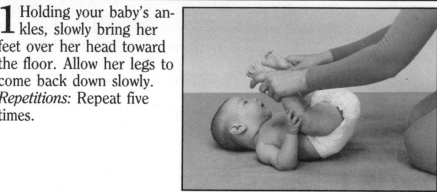

1 *Variation:* With your baby in the same starting position, raise her left hand above her head and raise her right foot toward her hand. Repeat five times on each side, alternating sides.

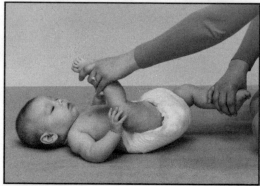

2 Bring both feet over the top of her head and hold for two seconds, then return to starting position. *Repetitions:* Repeat once.

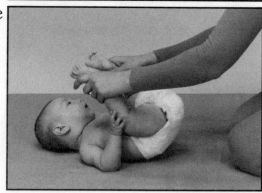

Note: Make a game of this exercise by peeking through your baby's legs while they are over her head.

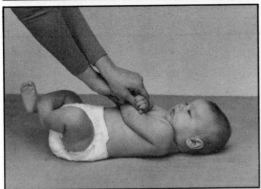

1 Holding your baby's hands, cross his left arm over his right arm, then cross his right arm over his left arm. *Repetitions:* Repeat three to five times with each arm, alternating arms.

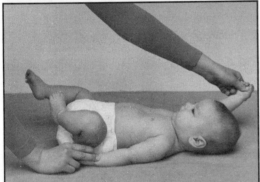

2 Raise his left arm above his head, then lower it to his side. Raise his right arm above his head, then lower it to his side. *Repetitions:* Repeat three to five times with each arm, alternating arms.

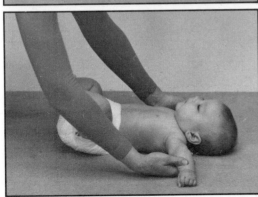

1 *Shoulder Rotations:* With your baby's arms at his sides and his palms facing up, hold his upper arms just above his elbows, then gently roll his arms until the palms of his hands are on the floor. Roll his hands back to starting position (i.e., with palms up). *Repetitions:* Repeat five times slowly.

Arm Stretching

Aim: To stretch your baby's arms and shoulders; a good warm-up exercise.

Starting Position: Lay your baby on his back.

Exercise No. 17

Leg Stretching

Aim: To loosen up your baby's leg muscles; a good warm-up exercise.

Starting Position: Lay your baby on his back.

1 Holding your baby's ankles, cross his left leg over his right leg, then cross his right leg over his left leg. *Repetitions:* Repeat three to five times with each leg, alternating legs.

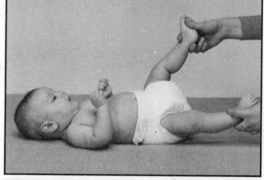

2 Raise his left leg above his head, then lower it. Raise his right leg above his head, then lower it. *Repetitions:* Repeat three to five times, alternating legs.

3 Holding onto your baby's ankles, slowly stretch his legs into a V.

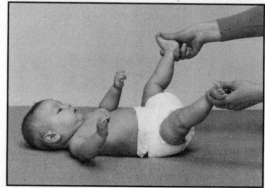

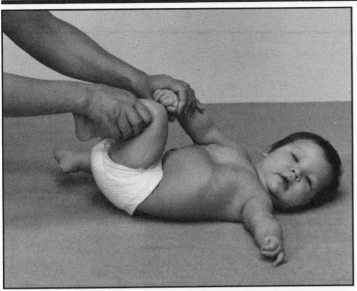

1 Raise her left knee while you bring her right hand down to slap her left knee lightly.

Knee Slappin'

Aim: To stretch your baby's body and improve her coordination.

Starting Position: Lay your baby on her back.

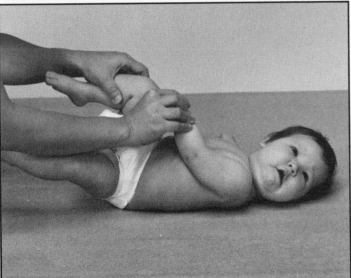

2 Raise her right knee and slap it with her left hand. *Repetitions:* Repeat five times on each side, alternating sides.

Exercise No. 19

1 Raise his left leg slightly, then gently cross it over his right leg until his toes touch the floor.

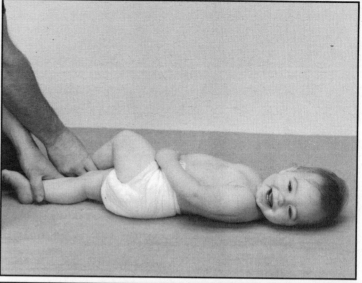

Baby Rainbows

Aim: To exercise your baby's entire leg; may help correct any tendency toward a "toed-in" walk.

Starting Position: Lay your baby on his back.

2 Roll his left leg outward to his left side, then return to starting position. Repeat with his right leg. *Repetitions:* Repeat five times on each leg, alternating legs.

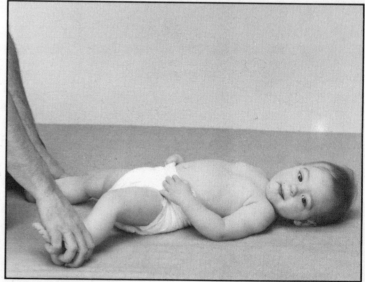

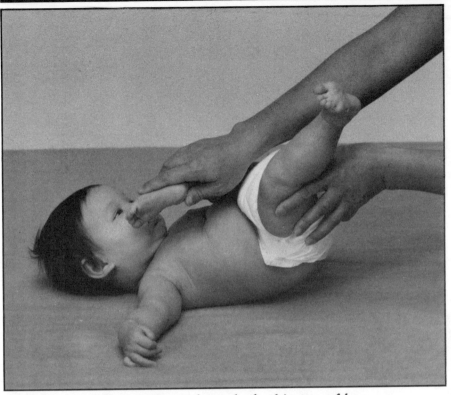

Touch Your Ear

Aim: To stretch your baby's entire body.

Starting Position: Lay your baby on her back.

1 Bring her left foot up, and touch the big toe of her left foot to her right ear. Touch the big toe of her right leg to her left ear. *Repetitions:* Repeat five to ten times on each side, alternating sides.

Exercise No. 21

Sitting

Aim: To prepare your baby for sitting, and to help develop the muscles he will use to pull himself to an upright position.

Starting Position: *Pull-ups:* Lay your baby on his back. *See-saws:* Sit on the floor with your legs apart and your baby lying on his back, facing you.

Note: When you do see-saws with your baby, say "up and down" to him as he moves, to help him recognize the concept of going up and down.

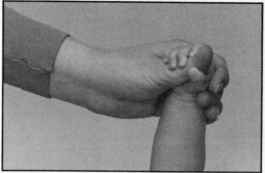

1 *Pull-ups:* Let your baby grasp your thumbs with both hands (Palmar grasp). Gently pull both of his arms upward, until you just begin to lift him off the floor.

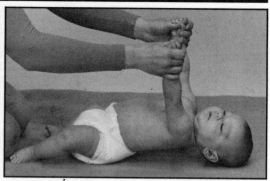

2 Keeping your hands very still at that position, allow your baby to pull himself up to your fingers. *Repetitions:* Repeat two or three times.

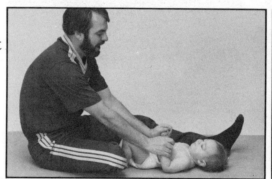

1 *See-saws (sit-ups):* Bend your right leg in and push your baby's legs against your right leg so that his legs are bent.

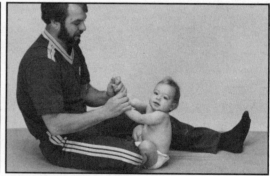

2 Have him grasp your thumbs, then wrap your hands around his and gently pull him up. Let him back down gently. If his head drops back when you pull him up, STOP the exercise. *Repetitions:* Start with five; work up to thirty.

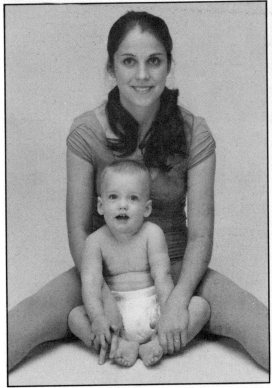

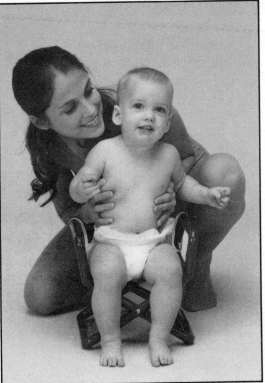

Sitting

Aim: To help your baby learn to sit by himself and to encourage good posture.

Starting Position: *Sitting on the Floor:* Sit on the floor with your legs apart. *Sitting on a Stool or Chair:* Place your baby on a chair or stacked mats.

1 *Sitting on the Floor:* Seat your baby between your legs, facing away from you while he rests against you. As your baby gains confidence, move back little by little until he is sitting by himself. *Do not* prop him up. Try letting him sit in a beanbag chair while you watch him.

1 *Sitting on a Stool or Chair:* Do not support your baby's back; give him a chance to balance on his own. To encourage him to keep his back straight, move a toy from side to side while he sits. For fun, play finger games with him while he sits.

Note: Until he is strong enough and confident enough to sit on his own, a four- to six-month-old baby can sit with your assistance for up to half an hour a day.

Exercise No. 22

Games on the Roll

Aim: To strengthen your baby's arms and legs for crawling.

Starting Position: Place a toy in front of a roll. Lay your baby on her stomach over the roll, holding her securely, keeping one hand on her back at all times.

Note: Use the *Strength Test* on page 145 to see whether your baby is ready for these exercises. Your baby should be at least four months old before you attempt Game #2 with her.

1 *Game #1:* Push your baby gently forward and backward for a minute or two. Allow the baby to use her legs to move the roll.

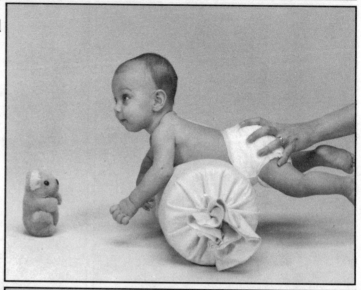

1 *Game #2:* Encourage your baby to grasp the toy on her own, allowing her to support her weight on her shoulders.

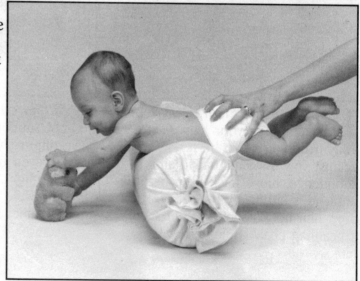

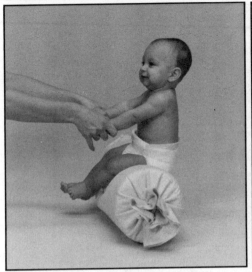 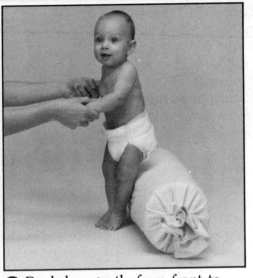

1 *Game #3 (Sitting to Stand):* Let your baby sit on the roll while you hold her hands firmly.

2 Rock her gently from front to back, moving her gradually to a stand. *Repetitions:* Repeat two or three times.

Games on the Roll

Aim: To improve your baby's balance and coordination.

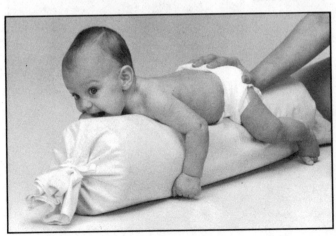

1 *Game #4 (Astride):* Place your baby lengthwise on her stomach on the roll, holding her tightly at the hips or thighs. Rock her from side to side, allowing her weight to fall on her hand and foot on each side. *Repetitions:* Rock her three to five times on each side.

157

Exercise No. 23

Crawling

Aim: To prepare your baby to support his weight on his shoulders and arms, prior to crawling.

Starting Position: *Pattern for Crawling:* Lay your baby on his back. *Wheelbarrow:* Place your baby on all fours, with his weight on his arms and shoulders. Hold his thighs with one hand while supporting his chest with the other.

1 *Pattern for Crawling:* Bend your baby's left knee toward his stomach and at the same time raise his right arm above his head. Return to starting position. *Repetitions:* Repeat five times on each side.

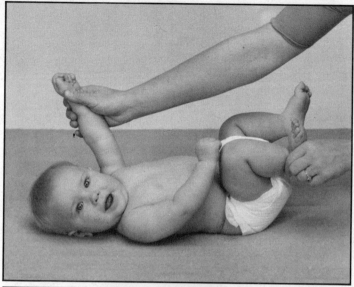

1 *Wheelbarrow:* Lift your baby's legs off the floor. Allowing him to support his own weight, "walk" him forward slowly on his hands for a very short distance. As he gets stronger, hold him at the knees—and, eventually, at the ankles—instead of at the thighs.

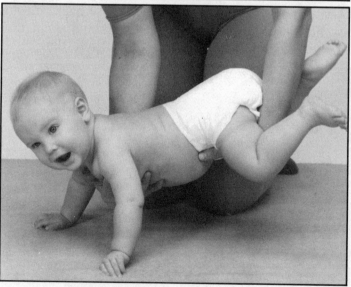

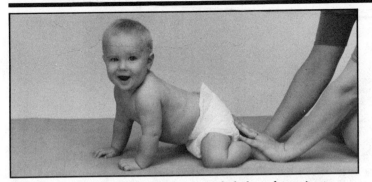

1 *Push and Creep:* Place your left hand against your baby's left foot and resist while he straightens his leg. Immediately place your right hand on his right foot. Alternate legs as he moves along the floor. At first he may have difficulty freeing his hand from under him. Let him try to pull his arm out, but be ready to help him.

Crawling

Aim: To strengthen your baby's legs and neck, to teach him how to reach, and to show him how to crawl properly.

Starting Position: *Push and Creep:* Place your baby on his stomach and tuck his feet up close to his body. *Fundamentals of Crawling:* Place your baby on all fours in a crouched position.

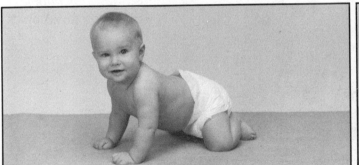

1 *Fundamentals of Crawling:* Rock your baby back and forth (revving). Eventually he will catch on to this rocking motion and do it himself, in preparation for crawling. Try placing a favorite toy in front of him for encouragement.

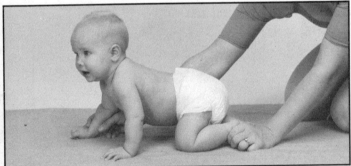

2 When your baby is ready, help him move his left knee and right arm forward at the same time. *Repetitions:* Repeat with his right knee and left arm; alternate as the baby crawls.

159

Exercise No. 24

Weight Lifting

Aim: To strengthen your baby's legs, develop her balance and eye/hand coordination, and teach her proper lifting techniques.

Starting Position: Stand behind her and hold her at the hips while she stands.

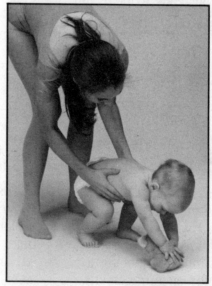

1 Encourage her to squat to pick up a toy or another object.

2 Return her to standing position. *Repetitions:* Repeat two or three times.

Note: Your baby must be able to stand on the floor fairly well before you attempt this exercise with her.

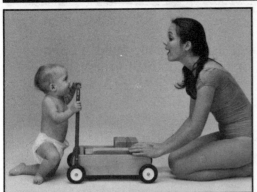

1 *Crawling to Stand:* Hold the push toy steady while your baby crawls up to it, pulls himself up, and uses it to walk. Eventually he will be able to push the toy by himself while you guide it.

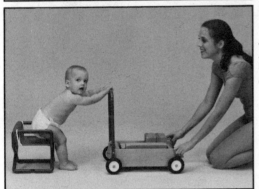

1 *Sitting to Stand:* Hold the push toy while your baby pulls himself to stand, out of the chair. Allow him to use the toy to walk holding onto the push toy.

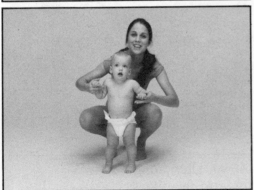

1 *Fundamentals of Walking:* Allow your baby to walk with your assistance, making sure that his feet are flat on the floor and his body is bent forward slightly. Practice for a few minutes at a time, until he is walking alone.

Walking

Aim: To prepare your baby for walking by giving him confidence to walk alone and to help your baby develop a natural stride.

Starting Position: *Crawling to Stand:* Seat your baby on the floor beside a push toy. *Sitting to Stand:* Seat your baby on a stool or baby seat beside a push toy. Hold your baby at the waist or hold his hands at waist level.

Exercise No. 1

Parents and baby will both benefit from the following exercises. Holding your baby while exercising increases resistance, which, for the parent, makes the exercises like exercising with weights. Start with a few exercises and increase the number as your family builds its fitness level. Try to add one or two a month to your baby's normal routine.

Roly-Poly

Aim: To massage your baby's back and loosen up your legs.

Starting Position: Pike sit. Place your baby across your legs, on her back.

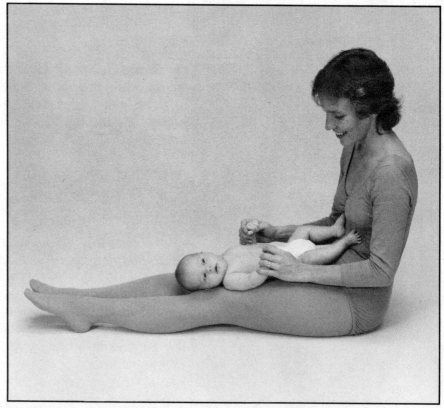

1 Move your thighs up and down, alternating legs. *Repetitions:* Repeat three to five times.

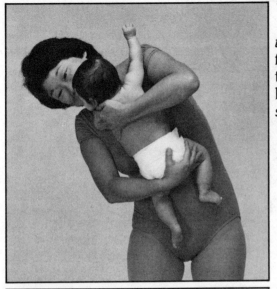

1 Bend to the left, then bend to the right. *Repetitions:* Begin by bending five times on each side, alternating sides; work up to bending ten times on each side.

Side Benders

Aim: To trim your waistline.

Starting Position: Stand with your legs apart, holding your baby in a tight hug, facing you.

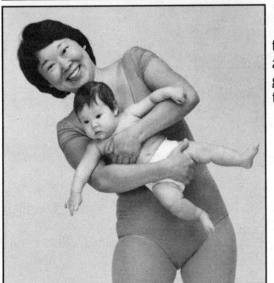

1 *Variation:* Do the exercise with your baby turned around, his back against your chest. As he grows older, he may prefer this position.

Sky Diver/ Parachute

Aim: To develop your baby's Landau reflex and parachute reflex (see page 131 for more information on reflexes).

Starting Position: Stand with your legs comfortably apart and your knees slightly bent, with your baby sitting between your legs. Place a small toy on the floor about a foot in front of you.

2 Gently swing her back and forth two to five times.

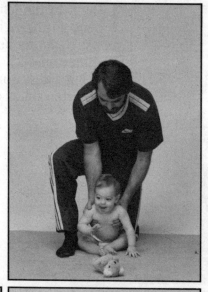

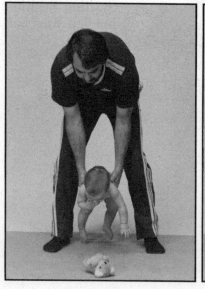

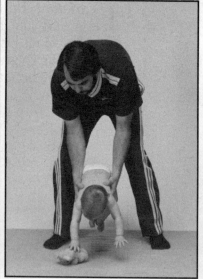

1 Squat down and pick up your baby, placing the palms of your hands on your baby's chest/stomach.

3 Tilt your baby so that her head points toward the floor; she will try to reach for the floor (parachute). *Repetitions:* Repeat two to five times. To strengthen your baby's grip, let her pick up a small object from the floor in front of you and raise it off the floor as high as she can.

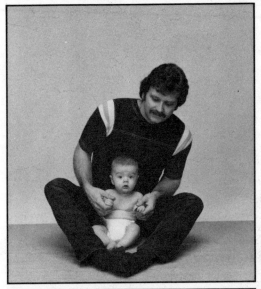

Butterfly Rock

1 Gently rock back and forth, then from side to side as you support your baby in your lap. *Repetitions:* Repeat five times.

Aim: To strengthen your inner thigh muscles and tone your legs and waist, and to tone your baby's thigh muscles.

Starting Position: You and your baby face in the same direction in the butterfly-sit position, with your baby's back against you.

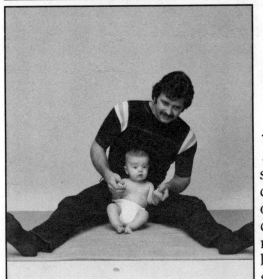

1 *Variation:* Try the exercise with you in a straddle-sit position. You can hold your baby's hands out at shoulder level in cross position to help him maintain his balance. Rock back and forth, then from side to side.

165

Exercise No. 5

Straddle Twist

Aim: To tone your baby's waistline.

Starting Position: Straddle sit, with your baby's back against your stomach, so that she is facing away from you.

1 Hold onto your baby's arms and gently twist her to the right, then the left, so that she moves from side to side at the waist. *Repetitions:* Repeat five times on each side; work up to ten.

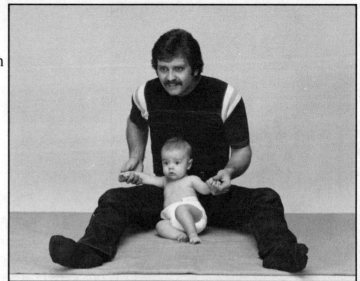

1 *Variation (Row-Row-Row Your Boat):* From the same starting position, hold onto your baby's arms and gently move them in a rowing or swimming position to the tune of "Row-Row-Row Your Boat."

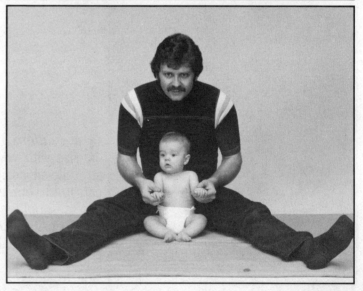

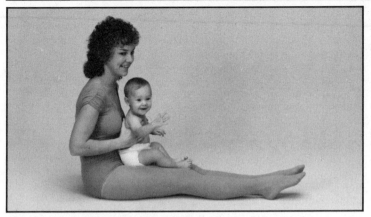

1 "Walk" forward with your seat and legs; do not use your heels. "Walk" backward in the same way.

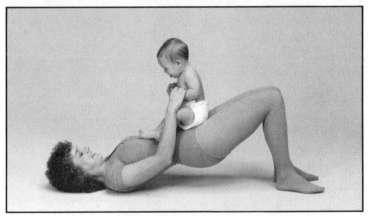

1 Raise your hips while you "tuck" your pelvis and pull in your abdominal muscles. Tighten your buttocks, then release the squeeze and lower yourself to starting position. *Repetitions:* Repeat five to ten times.

Ride Along
(team seat walks)

Aim: To tone your hips and legs.

Starting Position: Pike sit. Seat your baby on your lap with his back against you.

Note: For fun, put on a record while doing this exercise, and ride along with the beat of the song.

Ride 'em Baby
(team seat squeeze)

Aim: To strengthen your abdominal and pelvic muscles.

Starting Position: Hook-lying, with your baby sitting on your pelvic area facing you as you hold her around the waist.

Exercise No. 8

Porch Swing

Aim: To tone your waist and hips.

Starting Position: Hook-lying, with your baby sitting on your pelvic area facing you as you hold him around the waist.

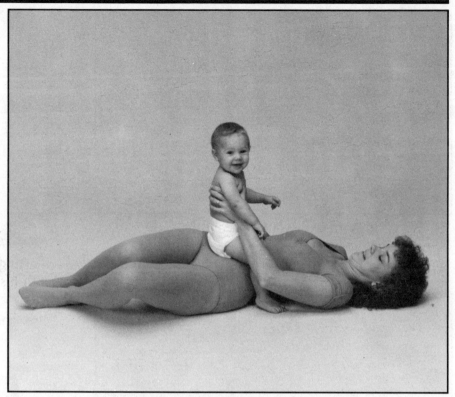

1 Keeping your shoulders and feet flat on the floor, roll your hips, dropping your knees to your left, then to your right side. *Repetitions:* Repeat five to ten times, alternating from side to side.

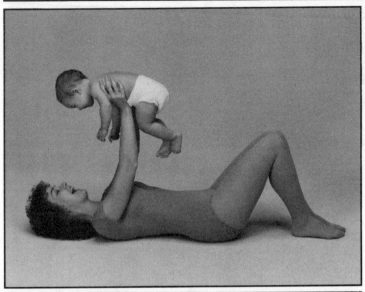

1 Holding your baby with your hands for balance, lift her until your arms are straight. Lower her to your chest. *Repetitions:* Repeat ten times.

Elevator

Aim: To strengthen your arms.

Starting Position: Lie on your back and lay your baby on your chest.

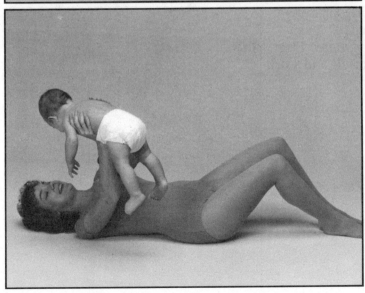

1 *Variations:* Holding your baby above your chest, move her in a circular motion, move her from side to side, and/or move her back and forth.

Exercise No. 10

Baby Curls

Aim: To strengthen your arms.

Starting Position: Stand, holding your baby in your arms.

1 Wrap one of your arms around your baby's legs and the other around his back, so that he is lying horizontally in your arms, parallel to the floor.

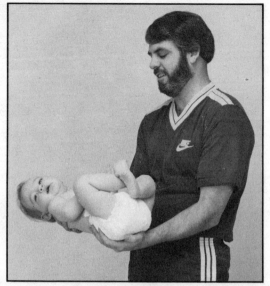

2 Slowly roll your arms open, then roll them back up. *Repetitions:* Start with two or three and work up to more.

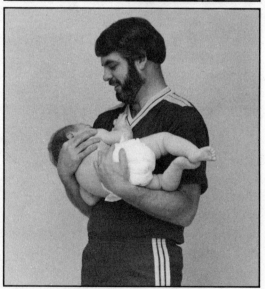

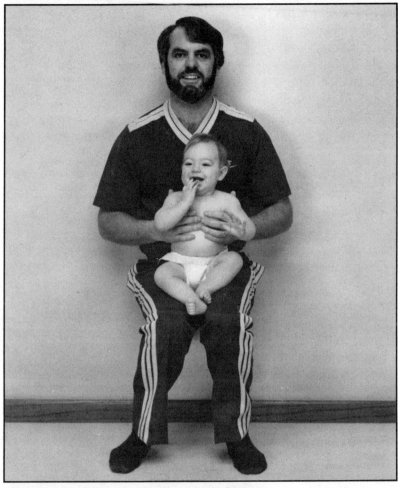

Skier's Sit

Aim: To strengthen your legs, abdominal muscles, and lower back.

Starting Position: Stand with your lower back pressed into the wall and your feet flat on the floor. Hold your baby with her back against your chest.

1 Slowly bend your knees until they are at approximately a ninety-five-degree angle to the wall (do not go any lower), as though you were sitting on a chair. Hold for five seconds or more, then slowly return to standing position. *Repetitions:* Repeat two to five times.

Exercise No. 12

See-Saws

Aim: To strengthen your baby's chest, hands, and arms.

Starting Position: *For babies two to four months old:* Hook-lying. *For babies four to twelve months old:* Straddle sit with your baby sitting on the floor between your legs, facing you.

Note: Use the Strength Test on page 145 to see if your baby is ready to try this exercise. When doing see-saws, say "up and down" to your baby as he moves, to help him recognize the concept of going up and down.

1 *For babies two to four months old:* Seat your baby on your stomach with his back against your thighs, facing you. Hold your baby's hands as you do sit-ups with him resting on your thighs. *Repetitions:* Repeat five to ten times.

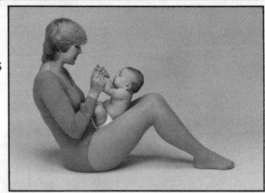

1 *For babies four to twelve months old:* Lay your baby on his back. Bend your right leg in and push his legs against your right leg so that his legs are bent.

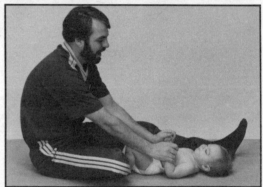

2 Have him grasp your thumbs (Palmar grasp), then wrap your hands around his and gently pull him up. Let him gently back down. If his head drops back when you pull him up, STOP the exercise; try again in a few weeks. *Repetitions:* Start with five sit-ups; work up to thirty.

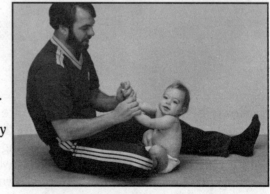

Exercise No. 13

1 Seat your baby on your shins, facing you and holding your hands. To a count of "One, two, three, wheel!" slide your feet up and down. Your head and shoulders will be slightly off the floor, but be sure your lower back remains pressed to the floor.

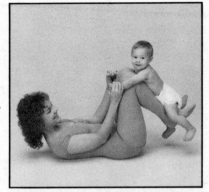

Knee Riders

Aim: To strengthen your abdominal muscles, shins, calves, and legs, and to strengthen your baby's legs.

Starting Position: Hook-lying.

1 *Giddy Up Baby:* Start in raised-knee-rider position, with your baby up in the air. Holding your baby under her arms, lower your feet and sit up so that she is sitting on the tops of your feet.

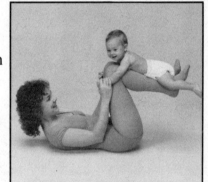
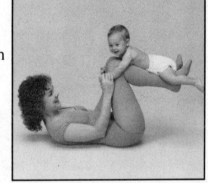

2 Alternate bending and extending your legs so that your baby moves in horse-riding fashion, kicking off from the floor.

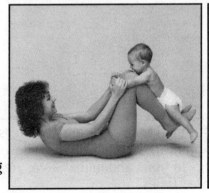
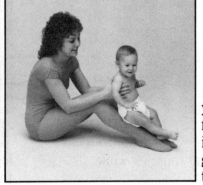

1 *Slides:* In hook-lying position, sit up and seat your baby on your knees, facing away from you. Holding her under the armpits, guide her down your shins to your feet.

173

Exercise No. 14

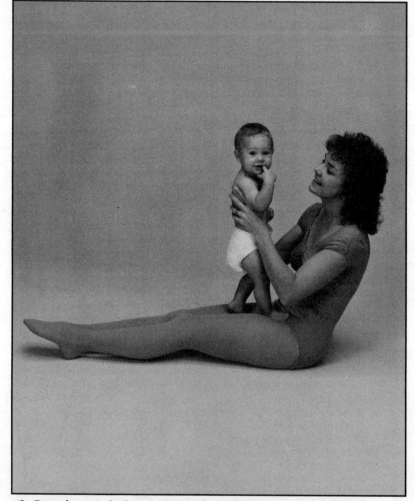

Tip-Toe through the Tulips

Aim: To strengthen your abdominal muscles.

Starting Position: Pike sit.

Note: Tighten your abdominal muscles while your baby walks up your legs.

1 Stand your baby on your legs, facing you. Holding him under his armpits, allow him to walk up your legs to your abdominal area. *Repetitions:* Repeat two to three times.

174

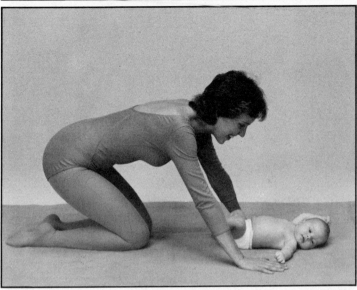

1 Rock forward, keeping your hands and knees in place.

Peck and Kiss

Aim: To strengthen your pectoral (chest) muscles, arms and shoulders.

Starting Position: Place your baby on her back on the floor and assume an all-fours position above her, with your hands near your baby's waist.

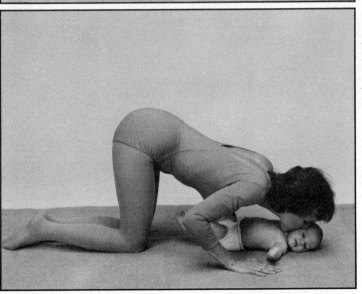

2 Bend your arms and lower your face to your baby's face, then plant a big kiss on her forehead. *Repetitions:* Repeat five to ten times.

Exercise No. 16

Baby Sweeps
(for both parents and baby)

Aim: To stretch your hamstrings.

Starting Position: You and your partner sit facing each other in straddle-sit position, with your feet touching. Place your baby between you and grasp your hands to form a circle around the baby.

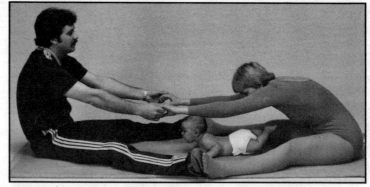

1 *Rowing:* Keeping your knees on the floor, gently lean backward, pulling your partner forward from the hips. Try to kiss the baby. *Repetitions:* You and your partner reverse roles and continue "rowing" back and forth five to ten times.

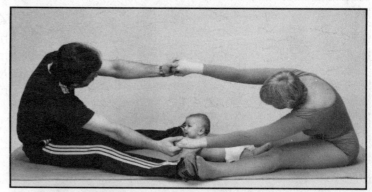

1 *Sweeps:* Starting from the same position, you and your partner "sweep" your upper bodies in a circular motion over your baby. *Repetitions:* Circle five times in each direction, alternating directions.

Exercise Mat

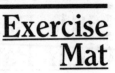

Materials:

• One piece of foam rubber, 5 feet × 24 inches × 1/2 inch.
• Two sections of coordinating calico print fabric, each 1-3/4 yards long.
• 72 inches of bias tape.

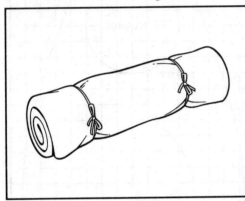

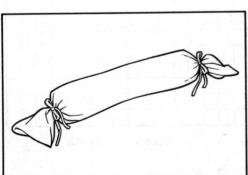

Directions:

1. Cut the cotton fabric into 1-3/4 yards × 26 inches (use the darker color for the bottom side).

2. Machine-applique YOU & ME, BABY in a solid color on the top fabric, right-side out.

3. Place the right sides together (wrong sides outside and showing) and sew along both sides and one end, giving a 5/8-inch seam allowance.

4. Turn the fabric right-side out, stuff foam into the casing, and adjust for even distribution.

5. Make ties by cutting two 36-inch pieces of bias tape. Zigzag stitch down the middle to finish off the ties.

6. Turn the bottom seam allowance on the mat in 5/8 inch and topstitch the edges together, placing bias tape ties in the seam at both ends. Secure the ties into the seam.

7. Roll up the mat, tie it, and you're ready to go.

Note: To make a baby exercise roll, roll up the mat and tie it at both ends.

To make a baby exercise roll that involves no sewing:

A suitable roll for these exercises can be made from a purchased foam bolster, 7 inches in diameter and 18 inches wide. You can cover it with toweling or colorful, washable fabric tied with ribbons on each end. As your baby gets older, add towels to adjust it to fit. The baby fits a roll when he can touch his hands in front of him and his feet are slightly off the floor behind him.

177

Little Beanbag Chair Pattern

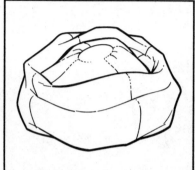

Materials:
- 3-1/2 yards of 45-inch or 3 yards of 60-inch material.
- Heavy-duty thread.
- Pellets to fill the chair.

Directions:

1. General notes: 1/2-inch seam allowances; sew all seams twice.

2. Cut one 9-inch circle, two 18-inch half circles, and six main pieces (see layout design).

3. Take two main pieces, place the right sides together, then stitch them and press the seam open. Continue to add the main pieces in like manner, until all six main pieces are sewn together, then join the first and last stitched pieces and stitch together to form a completed circle.

4. Place the 9-inch circle on top, matching the tops of the chair. Stitch, fitting in place as you sew.

5. Press under 1/2 inch on the raw edge of an 18-inch half circle. Sew the wrong sides of the circle together, leaving a seam opening of 5 inches.

6. Place the bottom circle and stitch it, fitting it as you sew it to the wrong sides. Then turn the chair right-side out and fill it with pellets.

7. Slipstitch the opening closed, very tightly.

Pattern

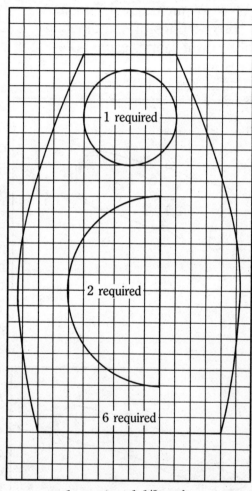

1 required

2 required

6 required

1 square = 1 1/2 yards

Appendix

Books

- Bing, Elisabeth. *Moving through Pregnancy* (Bantam).
- Levy, Janine, M.D. *The Baby Exercise Book* (Pantheon).
- Schneider, Virmala. *Infant Massage: A Handbook for Loving Parents* (Bantam).
- Simkin, Penny, R.P.T.; Whalley, Janet, R.N.; and Keppler, Ann, R.N. *Pregnancy, Childbirth, and the Newborn* (Meadowbrook).

Periodicals

American Baby, 575 Lexington Ave., New York, NY 10022.

Baby Talk, 185 Madison Ave., New York, NY 10016.

Growing Child/Growing Parent, 22 N. Second St., Lafayette, IN 47902.

Mothers Today, P.O. Box 243, Franklin Lakes, NJ 07417.

Parents, 80 New Bridge Rd., Bergenfield, NJ 07621.

The Physician and Sports Medicine, 4530 W. 77th St., Minneapolis, MN 55435.

Today's Health, American Medical Association, 535 N. Dearborn St., Chicago, IL 60610.

Organizations

American Medical Association
535 N. Dearborn St.
Chicago, IL 60610

American Running and Fitness Association
2420 K St. NW
Washington, DC 20037

Melpomene Institute for Women's Health Research
316 University Ave.
St. Paul, MN 55103

National Council of the YMCA of the USA
Director of Health Enhancement
101 N. Wacker Drive, Suite 1400
Chicago, IL 60606

YMCA of the USA, Program Resources
P.O. Box 5077
Champaign, IL 61820
(write for current catalog)

National Dairy Council
6300 N. River Rd.
Rosemount, IL 60018

American College of Obstetrics/Gynecology
600 Maryland Ave. SW, Suite 300 East
Washington, DC 20024

American Academy of Pediatrics
P.O. Box 1034
Evanston, IL 60204

Pregnancy Primer

Condition	Possible Causes	Possible Solutions
Backaches	Poor posture, enlarging uterus, loss of abdominal tone, incorrect body mechanics, body weight distribution, change in center of gravity, muscle tension due to stress, lack of flexibility, history of back problems (pathological or congenital), previous injuries, overused lumbar muscles.	Get a firm mattress, sleep on your side, exercise daily, avoid lifting and twisting, use proper posture techniques, wear low-heeled shoes, do pelvic rocking on back and all fours. Use proper lifting and bending techniques—avoid lifting anything higher than eye level, and lift only reasonable amounts, i.e., a maximum of one-fourth of your body weight (this is particularly a problem for women who have older children who want to be picked up for attention). Practice the tuck and pull exercise: "tuck" your pelvis and pull in your abdominal muscles.
Constipation	Hormonal changes cause your intestines to become sluggish, and your growing uterus displaces the intestinal tract.	Drink plenty of fluids, especially water; eat high-fiber foods, green leafy vegetables, grains. Get plenty of exercise. Avoid soda pop, caffeine, and alcohol.
Dizziness and Fainting Note: Notify your doctor if visual disturbances accompany dizziness or fainting.	Increased blood volume from pregnancy, decreased hemoglobin, low blood sugar.	Get up slowly; flex your ankles and bend your legs at the knees before getting up. Wear support stockings to promote better circulation to the upper part of your body (especially the brain). Eat protein-rich foods, not just carbohydrates, in the morning.
Edema (normal swelling of the extremities or face; not to be confused with metabolic edema or toxemia)	Retention of fluid.	Increase your water intake, elevate your legs, rest, and exercise. Consider water exercise as an alternative to "on land" exercise.

Pregnancy Primer

Condition	Possible Causes	Possible Solutions
Intestinal and Stomach Gas	Changes in body chemistry; physical pressure from the baby's growth causes decreased mobility of the intestinal tract, causing gas to form and the enlarging uterus to press on your intestines.	Avoid gas-producing foods; eat smaller, more frequent meals; and chew foods well. Exercise to increase intestinal activity—walking is especially good.
Headaches	Tension, stress, poor posture, poor circulation, diet, fatigue, eye strain.	Use total body relaxation techniques; take warm baths; try massage on upper body, neck, temples; do deep diaphragmatic breathing (don't hyperventilate). Stick to proper diet and use proper posture techniques. Get plenty of sleep (add ten percent to your normal sleep pattern, plus a nap in the afternoon).
Heartburn (uncomfortable burning sensation in the chest)	Acidic stomach secretions flow into your lower esophagus (most common in the second and third trimester). May be caused by the growing uterus pressing on your stomach.	Eat small, frequent meals; avoid alcohol, caffeine, acidic juices, spicy and gassy foods. Try proper diet selection. Change your position—try standing, sitting, lying down, or sleeping propped on pillows.
Hemorrhoids (varicose veins in the rectum)	Hemorrhoids are produced and aggravated by the pressure of the developing fetus. They may be aggravated further at the birthing stage of delivery, and by constipation.	Eat a diet high in fiber, do the kegel exercise, increase your water intake, do the pelvic rock exercise. Try a sitz bath or witch ha___ presses (to make your own c__ four-by-four compress ___ jar or dish, c__ refrig___
Insomnia	Movement of your b___ urination d___ em__	

Pregnancy Primer

Condition	Possible Causes	Possible Solutions
Nausea and Vomiting (a temporary condition experienced by approximately 60 percent of pregnant women.) Note: Severe vomiting can cause weight loss and upset in electrolyte (i.e., fluid) balance. Consult your physician if this occurs.	Hormonal changes, emotional factors.	Eat complex carbohydrates in dry form (e.g., unsalted crackers, Cheerios).
Shortness of breath	Growing uterus, decrease in lung capacity, weight gain.	Do deep breathing techniques, change body position, exercise—especially walking.
Stretch Marks (may occur on the stomach, legs, breasts, and hips)	Heredity, loss of skin elasticity, rapid and excessive weight gain.	Keep your weight under control. Most women can tolerate the stretch from the developing baby, but excessive rapid weight gain may exceed the capacity of the skin to expand, resulting in stretch marks. You may wish to keep the skin lubricated with petroleum jelly or lotions; the best time to apply them is before going to bed. Never use petroleum jelly or lotion prior to exercise, because they have a tendency to hold in body heat.
Urinary Problems	The pressure of your uterus causes a kink or pinch in the ureters.	Increase your water intake. Do not do kegels; this could worsen the problem. Note: If this condition persists, see your doctor.
Varicose Veins (veins that have become enlarged and engorged with blood, usually in the lower extremities and/or rectal area. Varicose veins that appear or worsen with pregnancy often will improve after the pregnancy.)	Heredity, increased blood volume during pregnancy, which puts more strain on blood vessels. The enlarging uterus presses on the vessel that runs to your legs, causing slower return of blood from the legs and more strain on veins in the legs and perineum.	Elevate your legs, pressing your feet gently to the wall, several times a day. Wear support hose, especially when exercising. Avoid any binding hose, socks or clothes. Cool down after exercising.

Index

INDEX

Pregnancy, Childbirth, and the Newborn

A complete guide for expectant parents

Pregnancy, Childbirth, and the Newborn is a thorough, yet easy-to-use, guide covering all aspects of pregnancy, childbirth, and newborn care. It explains the parental choices available, rather than preaching one philosophy, so you can be confident that you know the options and can choose intelligently. The easy-to-use format is organized for quick reference with charts, illustrations, and photographs. The book is written by three childbirth educators and has received acclaim from doctors, nurses, and educators. **Only $10.75 ppd.**

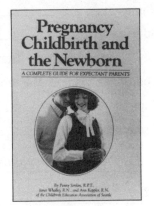

First-Year Baby Care

Edited by Paula Kelly, M.D.

The practical up-to-date guide for new parents. It's fully illustrated with over 100 step-by-step photographs and illustrations in a handy format. Dr. Paula Kelly includes what you want to know and what you need to know, from bathing and diapering to handling medical emergencies and baby development. It is authoritative yet practical and easy to use. The perfect companion for new parents. **Only $6.75 ppd.**

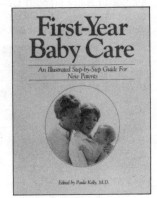

Parents' Guide To Baby & Child Medical Care

A first aid and home treatment guide that shows parents how to handle over 150 common childhood illnesses in step-by-step illustrated treatment format. Edited by Terril H. Hart, M.D., it contains: — *index of symptoms — record forms — height and weight charts — accident prevention — childproofing tips.* **Only $8.75 ppd.**

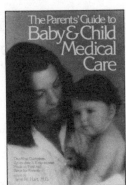

The Best Baby Name Book In The Whole Wide World

America's best-selling baby name book by Bruce and Vicki Lansky. More names, more up-to-date, more helpful, more entertaining, more gifty than any other baby name book! — *over 10,000 boys' and girls' names. . . more than any other book — how to name your baby: 15 rules — name psychology and stereotypes.* **Only $3.75 ppd.**

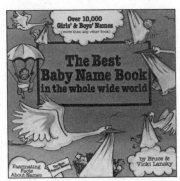

Our Baby's First Year

A colorful Baby Record Calendar that hangs on the nursery wall for handy use! OUR BABY'S FIRST YEAR is a "universal date" calendar plus a record book: 13 complete months for recording the "big events" of baby's first year as they happen. The day-by-day write-in spaces are undated, so OUR BABY'S FIRST YEAR starts whenever the baby arrives and lasts 13 months—a complete first year! For added convenience and color you can use the "baby's-firsts" stickers to mark the important milestones. Each month features a colorful baby animal nursery character to decorate the room, plus month-by-month development and baby care tips for quick reference. There's even a family tree and birth record form! A colorful and practical baby gift. **Only $9.50 ppd.**

My First Years

A beautiful baby record book to save your precious memories from arrival day to kindergarten! The colorful padded cover is reproduced from an original cross-stitch design of the *My First Friends* animals, with a delicate framing border. There are 32 pages of popular subjects like the family tree, a growth record, medical history, the first birthday, favorite photos, and many more. It is also gift boxed to be the perfect shower or new-arrival gift. **Only $11.75 ppd.**

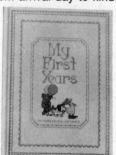

ORDER FORM

Name _____

Address _____

City _____ State _____ Zip _____

Charge ☐ Visa ☐ Mastercharge   Acct # _____

Expiration Date _____

Signature _____

Check or money order payable to Meadowbrook

Qty.	Title	Cost Per Book	Amount

We do not ship C.O.D. Postage and handling included in all prices.   **Total**

Your group or organization may qualify for group quantity discounts: please write for further information to Meadowbrook, 18318 Minnetonka Blvd., Deephaven, MN 55391

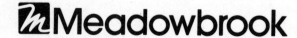

18318 Minnetonka Boulevard • Deephaven, Minnesota 55391